THE CORONARY CARE UNIT

APPLETON–CENTURY-CROFTS
EDUCATIONAL DIVISION/MEREDITH CORPORATION
NEW YORK

THE CORONARY CARE UNIT

WILLIAM J. GRACE, M.D.

Director
Department of Medicine
St. Vincent's Hospital and Medical Center
New York, New York

VICTOR KEYLOUN, M.D.

Department of Medicine
St. Vincent's Hospital and Medical Center
New York, New York

Copyright © 1970 by MEREDITH CORPORATION

740-1

Library of Congress Catalog Card Number: 74-110162

PRINTED IN THE UNITED STATES OF AMERICA
390-37940-9

*This book is dedicated to
the resident physicians, interns, and nurses of
Saint Vincent's Hospital and Medical Center
who made it possible.*

PREFACE

This is a book about the Coronary Care Unit. Our prime interest in presenting the subject is to describe the unit in terms of an organized system for managing patients with acute myocardial infarction. The book is intended as a guide for those who are starting or are about to start a CCU and is the result of our personal experience and second thoughts after supervising such a unit for the past five years. It is not intended to be a textbook of cardiology, although some aspects of the management of acutely ill patients with acute coronary artery disease are described in detail. The authors feel strongly that the establishment of a system of care for patients with acute myocardial infarction which includes the attitude of physicians, nurses, administration, and technicians; the localization of patients into groups; and the perfusion throughout the hospital of the concept of aggressive management of arrhythmia and cardiac resuscitation has proven that there is measurable benefit to the patients.

Considerable emphasis in this book is placed on the detection and the aggressive management of cardiac arrhythmias. This is the basic message we aim to convey. Emphasis is also placed on this aspect of acute myocardial infarction because the early detection and early treatment of these arrhythmias is frequently delegated to and must be attended to by the nonmedical staff. Less detail and attention is given to the phenomenon of shock and congestive heart failure, as these are more troublesome to deal with and the coronary care system in its present state probably contributes little to recovery from such complications.

A short, recent bibliography is included for further reading. It is not intended as a source of all references or all details. Interested readers can use these references for additional sources.

Some original concepts and aspects of coronary care are difficult to attribute. It is clear that the Coronary Care Unit concept in this country was pioneered by Hughes Day and Lawrence E. Meltzer, and by Kenneth W. G. Brown in Canada. Some particular phrases such as "life threatening arrhythmia" and "aggressive management" are very difficult to attribute. These phrases are so useful it is regrettable that we cannot give proper credit to their creator.

We must take this opportunity to express our gratitude to all the nurses who have worked so well on the CCU at St. Vincent's Hospital. We are especially grateful to Miss Patricia Fidgeon and Mrs. Mary Leone whose nursing skills are only surmounted by their patience. Without them we would not have such a unit, with them we have managed to create some order out of original chaos. Mrs. Jean McKinney, recently appointed head nurse to our Coronary Care Unit, has been of invaluable assistance.

We wish to thank Sister M. Eileen Hawkey, Director of Nursing Service at St. Vincent's Hospital, and Miss Rita Rowland for their invaluable advice and assistance over many years. Mr. Albert J. Samis, our associate administrator, has given sound advice and counsel over these years and for this we are very grateful.

We are especially proud of the role our house staff has played in patient care since the beginning of our Coronary Care Unit and want to take this opportunity to express our gratitude to them. Dr. William Minogue and Dr. Victor Keyloun were Chief Medical Residents when our unit was started. Dr. Stephen Ayres and his special knowledge of pulmonary physiology has not only saved lives and stopped arrhythmias, but has also been a constant source of help in problem-solving and a most substantial aide in all of the work involved in setting up and maintaining our Coronary Care Unit. Dr. John J. Gregory, in addition to many other things, has inserted practically all of the temporary transvenous electric pacemakers and deserves our gratitude.

The help and cooperation of our EKG technicians can be used as a model for any institution. We are forever grateful to Miss Claire McMann for her leadership, loyalty, and competence.

Finally, we wish to express our gratitude to Dr. Richard J. Kennedy, Associate Director of Medicine and Chief of Cardiology at St. Vincent's Hospital, for his constant support, help, and expertise.

The photographs used in this text were prepared by Mr. Rudolf Henning of St. Vincent's Hospital.

CONTENTS

THE CORONARY CARE UNIT

1

The Natural History of Patients with Acute Myocardial Infarction

The Magnitude of the Problem

Coronary artery disease is the leading cause of death in the United States today. Among males in the prime of life, it is of epidemic proportions. This is shown graphically in Figure 1. Over 500,000 persons die of coronary disease every year. It is estimated that 1,500,000 episodes of acute myocardial infarction occur per year in the United States. Only half of the 500,000 who die of this condition reach a hospital. Of those patients who reach a hospital the mortality rate is very high, from 30 to 40 percent. This represents a national health problem of staggering proportions. A reduction of the mortality rate by merely 10 percent would return at least 50,000 men to useful and productive lives.

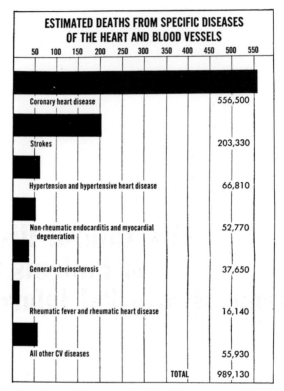

Fig. 1. A recent tabulation of the cause of death (From the National Center for Health Statistics, 1965).

The Day of Death

Data from many studies indicate that the hospital mortality rate is highest on the first day and less on the second and third days, and that practically all hospital deaths occur in the first hospital week (Fig. 2). It is inferred from this information that a given patient with an acute myocardial infarction who reaches a hospital is at the time of greatest risk from the first to the fifth day of his illness. The clinical episode of acute myocardial infarction may be considered to be associated with a period of crisis which the patient may not survive. If he does survive the first few crucial days a favorable outcome is likely.

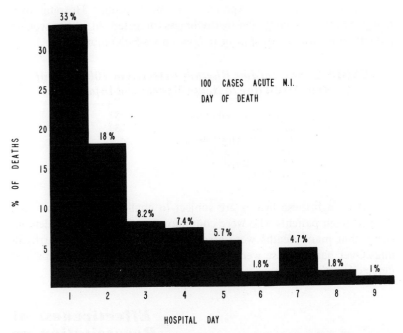

Fig. 2. A tabulation of 100 deaths at St. Vincent's Hospital from acute myocardial infarction. In this series of patients autopsies were performed on 44 percent. Note that at 5 days, 73 percent of the deaths have occurred.

Mechanism of Death

An analysis of the causes of death in acute infarction from various institutions and different series shows causes that are predictable from year to year. Although pulmonary embolism and rupture of the ventricle account for some of the deaths, most are associated with disorders and mechanisms that are, theoretically at least, treatable, such as arrhythmia, shock, and congestive heart failure. Table 1, based on data from premonitoring times at St. Vincent's Hospital, is probably reasonably accurate. Note that almost half of the deaths were due to cardiac arrhythmia.

TABLE 1. *Cause of Death in Acute Myocardial Infarction*

Arrhythmia	40%
Shock	20%
Congestive Heart Failure	20%
Others	20%

Table 2, based on experience at St. Vincent's Hospital over many years, indicates the arrhythmias detected in the coronary patient with cardiac arrest prior to continuous ECG monitoring.

TABLE 2. *The Cardiac Rhythm Detected in 108 Cases of Cardiac Arrest due to Acute Myocardial Infarction*

Ventricular Fibrillation	51
Asystole	32
Complete Heart-Block	9
Sinus Bradycardia	3
Chaotic Rhythm	11
No ECG	2

Although these figures are subject to challenge, as they are not derived from patients who were continuously monitored, they demonstrate that many deaths were associated with "correctable" arrhythmias.Over half of these were treatable and theoretically correctable if detected in time.

Effectiveness of Resuscitation on Mortality in Acute Myocardial Infarction

Analysis of our experience shows that the common denominator of success in resuscitation is the presence of a physician and the availability of the necessary equipment to restore normal rhythm. If one considers all attempts at resuscitation the success rate is indicated in Table 3.

TABLE 3. *Results of Resuscitation—Effect of Time Lag*

Physician Immediately Available	
Permanent Survivors	14 (22%)
Fatalities	50
	64
Physician Not Immediately Available	
Permanent Survivors	1 (2%)
Fatalities	43
	44

Basis for the Coronary Care Unit

A consideration of the preceding data leads to the inevitable conclusion that myocardial infarction is associated early in the course of illness with life-threatening arrhythmias which, if detected, are treatable. It seems clear that to perform this service patients with acute myocardial infarction must be segregated in a special area of the hospital where their ECG can be continuously monitored and early signs of impending life-threatening arrhythmias may be detected and treated. They must be cared for by a specially trained staff, immediately available, experienced in the technique of cardiac resuscitation, and convinced of the worth of the concept of "aggressive" management of arrhythmias in acute myocardial infarction.

Variations in Mortality Rates in Patients with Acute Myocardial Infarction

We reviewed 596 charts of patients discharged from our hospital with a diagnosis of acute myocardial infarction during two consecutive years (1965 and 1966). Autopsies were performed on 44 percent of the fatal cases. Of these patients, 114 were excluded from the study because detailed evaluation of the hospital course, serial electrocardiograms, and serum enzymes revealed no evidence of acute myocardial infarction. This state might be called the "coronoid" syndrome, for the patients had symptoms suggestive of acute myocardial infarction, but confirmatory tests did not substantiate this diagnosis. In about half of these patients there seemed to be no acute illness. In the remainder the diagnoses of heart failure, pulmonary edema, pulmonary embolus, or esophagitis, with or without "old" myocardial infarction, seemed adequate to account for the symptoms.

There were 106 patients with a condition classified as "subendocardial" infarction. For want of a better name, we have come to call this the "coronette" syndrome. The clinical syndrome consisted of mild to severe chest pain. The serial electrocardiograms revealed slight to moderate changes in the T waves only; enzyme changes if present were moderate. In patients with this condition there was no mortality, except for three who died of other causes (gangrene of feet, cerebrovascular accident, and pulmonary embolus); autopsy in two of these patients revealed normal coronary arteries and no myocardial infarction.

Patients with what we call a "coronary" had acute transmural myocardial infarction, as indicated by significant Q wave patterns in the electrocardiogram and sequential S-T and T wave changes. There were 368 such patients. In this group, serum glutamic oxalacetic transaminase (SGOT) and lactic dehydrogenase (LDH) levels were at least twice normal. Serum creatinine phosphokinase (CPK) levels were elevated in all cases to twice the normal level. When patients were admitted with pre-existing abnormal electrocardiograms, the diagnosis of acute myocardial infarction was excluded unless the CPK level was significantly elevated. In this manner an attempt was made to separate patients with pulmonary edema and less serious but mimicking conditions from those with myocardial infarction. The serum CPK level has been found to be very reliable in diagnosing myocardial infarction. Besides the heart, only skeletal muscle and brain tissue contain CPK in quantities sufficient to elevate serum levels. Serum GOT and LDH may be elevated in pulmonary edema because of passive congestion of the liver, but the serum CPK will be elevated only if myocardial necrosis has occurred.

Mortality Rate in Acute Transmural Myocardial Infarction

On the basis of these criteria we have limited our consideration of mortality to acute transmural infarction and to several variables that influence the outcome. These variables are subdivided as follows:

I. Degree of acute left ventricular dysfunction.
   A. no left ventricular dysfunction;
   B. moderate congestive heart failure or hypotension (90 mm Hg systolic or less);
   C. shock or acute pulmonary edema.

II. Age.

Further classification is made according to age. A varying mortality rate clearly related to age and the severity of left ventricular dysfunction is indicated. (See Tables 4, 5 and 6.)

III. Pre-existing complications in patients.

The presence of concomitant disease definitely increases the mortality rate. Therefore, in considering the mortality rate, patients with the diagnosis of acute myocardial infarction should be further classified according to the presence of one or more of the following conditions:

  A. diabetes;
  B. hypertension;
  C. previous acute myocardial infarction;
  D. no complications.

In the following tables the "mortality" rate indicates the hospital mortality at St. Vincent's Hospital. The "range" is the mortality rate in the combined hospital collected series of the USPHS, also with continuous cardiac monitoring. At this time there are a combined total of 2,174 patients from all sources.

TABLE 4. *Acute Transmural Myocardial Infarction Mortality Rate*

AGE	MORTALITY SVH STUDY	RANGE REPORTED SERIES IN USPHS STUDY
55 or less	9%	(8–25%)
56 to 64	21%	(17–31%)
65 and over	37%	(30–47%)

Based on 2,174 patients in USPHS study.

TABLE 5. *Acute Myocardial Infarction Mortality Rate*

	MORTALITY SVH STUDY	RANGE REPORTED SERIES IN USPHS STUDY
Class A	17%	(10– 22%)
Class B	38%	(33– 55%)
Class C	72%	(70–100%)

TABLE 6. *Mortality Rate by Age Groups and Class of Ventricular Dysfunction, January 1965 to June 1966*

Transmural Myocardial Infarction Only

AGE	55 OR LESS	56-65	OVER 65	TOTAL
Class A	9%	23%	50%	27%
Class B	33%	50%	42%	42%
Class C	66%	91%	90%	88%
Total	14%	33%	53%	

The variables included under acute left ventricular dysfunction, age and coexistent disease(s), place a patient in one of 72 possible categories for mortality evaluation.* Hence, it is apparent that unless large numbers of patients are studied and all variables considered little significant information will be reported.

TABLE 7. *Acute Myocardial Infarction Mortality Rate* [*Total Patients—397*]

Effect of Pre-Existing Complication—SVH Series

		ALIVE	DEAD
Diabetes	(57)	29	28
Previous AMI	(72)	34	38
Hypertension	(56)	41	15
None of above	(212)	156	56

Further variability in reported mortality rates will be accounted for if one considers the interval of time between the onset of the pain and time of hospitalization (Fig. 3). For example, the occurrence of ventricular fibrillation is an early event in the course of acute myocardial infarction, indeed most of it occurring in the first few hours. The data in Table 8 indicates this clearly.

* The figure 72 is arrived at by using the following formula: $[3 \times 3] [1 + (2^n) - 1]$ where $[3 \times 3] =$ age x class; $1 =$ no disease; and $n =$ number of associated diseases.

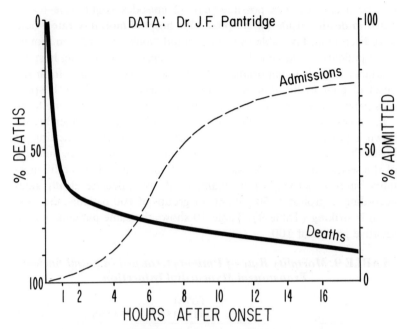

Fig. 3. Death occurs within the first hour after the onset of chest pain in over half the cases. Admissions to the hospital peak between 4 and 8 hours after the onset of pain. It is apparent that most of the deaths occur before the patient reaches the hospital.

TABLE 8. *Primary Ventricular Fibrillation*

Patients with Acute Myocardial Infarction (Transmural)	625
Patients with Primary Ventricular Fibrillation	85

In Coronary Care Unit (CCU)	44
In Emergency Room (E.R.)	32
	76*

% Overall Survivors	68%

% Survivors in CCU	41%
% Survivors in E.R.	75%

* *Nine patients had V.F. in other parts of hospital.*

In our hospital, most patients with acute myocardial infarction are admitted within 4 to 6 hours of the onset of the pain. If admission had been delayed it is possible that 32 episodes might have terminated in death outside the hospital. Our hospital mortality rate would have been more favorable to us and would "look" better, even though more patients would actually have died. Hence, in evaluating hospital mortality rates it is important to know the interval of time from the onset of pain to the time of arrival at medical care. If the hospital sees patients early in this disease, ventricular fibrillation is going to be a more common complication. Even with this spread, further breakdown is possible and probably necessary if one considers the time of hospitalization, sex of the patient, location of the infarction, and size of the series. In the last instance, marked variability of "overall" mortality rates is striking. For example, if we calculate death rates according to groups of 50 patients or groups of 100 patients, the variation is striking (Table 9). Table 10 shows the same patients in consecutive groups of 100.

TABLE 9. *Mortality Rate of Patients Grouped in Small Series:*
Transmural Myocardial Infarction

	TOTAL PATIENTS*	DEATHS	RATE
January 1965 to May 1965	48	11	21%
June 1965 to September 1965	55	6	10%
October 1965 to December 1965	44	19	44%
January 1966 to March 1966	54	16	24%
April 1966 to July 1966	51	9	17%

Listed in consecutive groups of approximately 50 patients.

TABLE 10. *Mortality Rate of Patients Grouped in Large Series:*
Transmural Myocardial Infarction

	TOTAL PATIENTS*	DEATHS	RATE
January 1965 to September 1965	103	17	16%
October 1965 to March 1966	98	35	35%

* *Listed in consecutive groups of approximately 100 patients.*

The considerations set forth here emphasize many of the pitfalls in the reporting of mortality rates of acute myocardial infarction, pitfalls such as a restrictive classification or an all-inclusive classification that embraces such entities as "subendocardial infarction," which notably has the effect of reducing any mortality rate. Other classifications of patients, depending upon complications (e.g., diabetes), also must be taken into consideration if one is to achieve a true estimate of mortality from myocardial infarction. It should be considered as a disease entity in itself, or one associated with, or influenced by, other conditions. The variability in "overall" mortality rate reflects the importance of age and preexistent complicating diseases.

Mortality Outside the Hospital

It is estimated from various sources that a substantial number of deaths from acute myocardial infarction occur before the patient is able to reach medical care. The following table substantiates this:

TABLE 11. *Coronary Deaths; North London**

Before Ambulance Arrived	47%
In Ambulance	13%
In Hospital	40%

* Data from Pantridge, 1967.

This information is diagrammatically demonstrated in the following graph taken from Pantridge and Geddes (Fig. 3).

The data clearly indicate that many, if not half, of such deaths occur before the patient receives medical care, because of the system in which we now live. Such things are well known to the lay public, and even casual examination of the daily newspapers will indicate that a large number of people "died at home" or "dropped dead on the street." A few typical newspaper clippings emphasize this point.

Mark Shaw, the White House photographer for President Kennedy, died of a heart attack Sunday night in his apartment at 343 East 30th Street. He was 47 years old.—*New York Times*, Tuesday, January 28, 1969

Williston Park—Peter Franconi, 63, who died last Monday while shoveling snow in front of his Williston Park home, was the plant electrical engineer at Reeves Instrument Corp. at Roosevelt Field. An obituary in *Newsday* on Friday incorrectly identified Franconi as a tailor.—*Newsday*, Monday, February 17, 1969

Crowd strains to get glimpse of Royal Little's winning performance in first-race win on Big A's opening day. Some won, some lost—and some died yesterday as Aqueduct racetrack opened a new season. Three men, one a track employee, collapsed and died at the track. "There's nothing unusual about this," one policeman said. "They just got overexcited. We normally have one or two die on the first day of racing."—*New York Daily News*, Tuesday, March 11, 1969

Mechanism of Cardiac Arrest in "Sudden" Death

Such deaths are presumed to be due to arrhythmias, rather than shock, pulmonary edema, or rupture of the ventricle. The data on the early incidence of arrhythmias are somewhat scarce, although the recent publication of Pantridge is quite convincing. He showed in a recent study that over half of the patients with inferior infarction had bradyarrhythmia, A-V dissociation, or complete heart block. These are patients seen within an hour of the onset of the acute myocardial infarction by his Mobile Coronary Care Unit. Such a high occurrence of bradyarrhythmia is quite different from the frequencies of bradyarrhythmia seen in the hospitalized patient, and it is Pantridge's feeling that these arrhythmias cause the largest number of deaths that occur outside the hospital.

The advent of the coronary care unit has substantially reduced the mortality in hospitalized patients, and most institutions, including our own, are reporting reductions from a former rate of 35 percent to a current rate of 18 to 20 percent. This improvement, of course, applies only to the patient who has reached the hospital.

If we are to reduce further the mortality rate from myocardial infarction, then the Coronary Care Unit must be brought to the patient so that the safeguards it affords are available to him sooner than they are at the present time. This is the basic concept of the Mobile Coronary Care Unit of Pantridge which, on receiving a call, brings to the patient's bedside, or to his factory, office, or home, a team of physicians and the battery-driven components of an intensive care-coronary care unit.

Concluding Remarks

A study of the natural history of the patient with acute myocardial infarction indicates a very high mortality rate on the first hospital day and a decreasing mortality rate on the second and third hospital days. If the patient can survive the first few days, a time of crisis, then the outlook is reasonably good. During these critical first few days, patients die of congestive heart failure, of shock, and of life-threatening arrhythmias. The last can be controlled by suitable and appropriate medication or electrical means if promptly detected. It is in this area that the greatest hope of therapy lies at the present time, and on this concept the Coronary Care Unit has evolved. Table 12 shows the changing mortality at St. Vincent's Hospital since instituting the Coronary Care Unit (1964).

TABLE 12. *Acute Myocardial Infarction: Mortality Rate*

	ALIVE	DEAD	CCU TOTAL	HOSP. DEAD*
1964	119	56	N/A	32%
1965	100	34	134	26%
1966	132	50	182	27%
1967	142	31	173	17%

* Excludes death in Emergency Room. All patients had transmural myocardial infarction.

References

Adgey, J., Geddes, J. S., Mulholland, H. C., Keegan, D. A. J., and Pantridge, J. F. Incidence, significance & management of early bradyarrhythmias complicating acute myocardial infarction. Lancet, 2:1097, 1968.

Anderson, I. W., le Richie, W. H., and MacKay, J. S. Sudden death: Correlation with hardness of water supply. New Eng. J. Med., 280:80, 1969.

Day, H. W. Acute coronary care—A Five Year Report. Amer. J. Cardiol., 21:252, 1968.

———— Effectiveness of an intensive coronary care area. Amer. J. Cardiol., 15:51, 1965.

Early care of coronary subject. Sixth Bethesda Conference. Amer. J. Cardiol., 23:603, 1969.

Goble, A., Sloman, G., and Robinson, J. S. Mortality reduction in a coronary care unit. Brit. Med. J., 1:1005, 1966.

Grace, W. J. The use of monitoring devices in acute myocardial infarction. Adv. in Cardiopulm. Dis., 4:91, 1969.

———— Mortality rate from acute myocardial infarction. What are we talking about? Amer. J. Cardiol., 20:301, 1967.

———— Use of a Coronary Care Unit for Patients with Acute Myocardial Infarction, Rheumatic and Coronary Disease. A Medical Surgical Symposium sponsored by St. Barnabas Hospital, New York, J. B. Lippincott Co., 1967.

———— and Chadbourn, J. A. The mobile coronary care unit. Dis. Chest, 55:452, 1969.

———— and Soscia. J. L. Reducing mortality from acute myocardial infarction—current ideas. Cardiol. Digest, 4:29, 1969.

Kannel, W. R., Barry, P., and Dawber, T. R. Immediate mortality in coronary heart disease. The Framingham study. Proc. 4th World Cong. Cardiol., 3:176, 1963.

Killip, T. III, Kimball, J. T. Treatment of myocardial infarction in a coronary care unit. A two year experience with 250 patients. Amer. J. Cardiol., 20:457, 1967.

Kuller, L., Lilienfeld, A., and Fisher, R. Epidemiological study of sudden and unexpected deaths due to arteriosclerotic heart disease. Circulation, 34:1056, 1966.

MacMillan, R. L., Brown, K. W. G., Peckham, G. B., Kahn, O., Hutchison, D. B., and Paton, M. Changing perspectives in coronary care. A five year study. Amer. J. Cardiol., 20:451, 1967.

Meltzer, L. E. Concepts and systems for intensive coronary care. Acad. Med. New Jersey Bull., 10:304, 1964.

Minogue, W. F., Smessart, A. A., and Grace, W. J. External cardiac massage for cardiac arrest due to myocardial infarction: a changing concept. Amer. J. Cardiol., 13:25, 1964.

Norris, R. M., Brandt, P. W. T., Caughey, D. E., Lee, A. J., and Scott, P. J. A new coronary prognostic index. Lancet, 1:274, 1969.

———— Brandt, P. W. T., and Lee, A. J. Mortality in a coronary care unit analysed by a new coronary prognostic index. Lancet, 1:278, 1969.

Pantridge, J. F., and Geddes, J. S. A mobile intensive care unit in the management of myocardial infarction. Lancet, 2:271, 1967.

Partamian, J. O., and Bradley, R. F. Acute myocardial infarction in 258 diabetics: immediate mortality and five-year survival. New Eng. J. Med., 273:455, 1965.

Sloman, G., Stannard, M., and Goble, A. J. Coronary care unit: a review of 300 patients monitored since 1963. Amer. Heart J., 75:140, 1968.
Sniekerman, R. E., Brandenburg, J. T., Achor, R. W. P., and Edwards, J. E. The spectrum of coronary heart disease in a community of 30,000: a clinicopathologic study. Circulation, 25:57, 1962.

2

The Coronary Care Unit: Design, Equipment, and Staff

In the preceding chapter it was shown that the patient with acute myocardial infarction is at the period of greatest risk for at least five to seven days following the onset of the attack, and that a great proportion of the deaths in this interval are due to treatable arrhythmias. In order to deal effectively with this problem, a number of people developed the concept of the Coronary Care Unit almost simultaneously in the United States and Canada; notable among them were Dr. Hughes Day at the Bethany Hospital in Kansas, Dr. Kenneth W. G. Brown at the Toronto Medical Center, and Dr. Lawrence E. Meltzer at University of Pennsylvania Presbyterian Hospital and Medical Center, Philadelphia. The original aim of the Coronary Care Unit was early detection of cardiac arrest and prompt resuscitation.

Historical Notes

Resuscitation, consisting of closed chest cardiac massage, electric defibrillation, and mechanical ventilation, is a procedure applied to the pulseless, non-breathing patient for the purpose of restoring the circulation. The concept of resuscitation goes back far in medical history, as indicated by the following:

> Where, however, the cessation of vital action is very complete we ought to inflate the lungs and pass electric shocks through the chest. Practitioners ought never, if death has been sudden and the person not very far advanced in life to despair of success . . .—Allen Burns, 1809, Glasgow

> For one seemingly killed with lightning, or suffocated, plunge him immediately into cold water, or, blow strongly with bellows down his throat. This may recover a person seemingly drowned. It is still better, if a strong man blows into the mouth.—*Primitive Physic*, John Wesley (1703-1791)

In spite of this early interest in resuscitation, little was accomplished in clinical medicine.

In the 19th century there were several isolated reports of resuscitation based on the experimental animal, using open chest cardiac massage. In 1829 Leroy-d'Etiolles advocated a method of artificial respiration involving pressure on the sternum:

> By this maneuver the stagnant blood in the vessels of the abdomen and chest is set in motion toward the heart and lungs; the contractility of the diaphragm returns; the contraction of the muscle infrequent and convulsive at first, soon becomes more and more regular: life returns.

Further explanation and clarification of this concept shows that he apparently did not appreciate the physiology of the maneuver as we know it today.

In 1891 Maass described closed chest cardiac massage in man such as it is known and performed today:

> One steps to the left side of the patient facing his head, and presses deep in the heart region with strong movements, while the heel of the opened right hand is placed between the site of

the apex beat and the left sternal border. The frequency of
compression is 120 or more per minute. The effectiveness of
the movement is recognized from the artificially produced
carotid pulse and the constriction of the pupils.

Modern therapy has modified this procedure very little; the
hand is placed over the lower one-third of the sternum and the rapid-
ity of compression decreased to about 60 to 70 per minute.

In this country, as early as 1904, George Crile described a successful resuscitation of cardiac arrest after thyroidectomy, employing
closed chest cardiac massage and epinephrine infusion. Other
attempts were made, but without success, and little attention was paid
to the event. These and other historical milestones lay unnoticed until
1960, when interest was reawakened by the work of Kouwenhoven.
In the 1930's Kouwenhoven investigated the electrical properties of
the heart and the use of the electric defibrillator for ventricular fibrillation. This, at first, was used sporadically in man, but in 1947 Beck
described the first successful resuscitation in the human from ventricular fibrillation by the use of electric countershock. The subject of
this modern-day miracle was a middle-aged physician. By 1954 thirty
cases of ventricular fibrillation were reported occurring during cardiac
surgery. Twenty of these hearts were defibrillated, and nine patients
recovered completely.

Successful resuscitation was at first a function of the speed with
which the physician delivered his therapy. The surgeon and anesthesiologist were best equipped in terms of availability to deliver this
therapy, as most of the cases of cardiac arrest which were thought to
be reversible occurred in the operating room. However, it was known
from the teaching of Claude Beck that during myocardial infarction
there were hearts "too good to die." He was the first to demonstrate
that successful resuscitation could take place outside the operating
room, but it was left to the insight of Hughes Day and others to bring
together all the elements necessary for resuscitation—to segregate
patients with similar illnesses for the more effective application of the
principles of therapy which had been known for over a century. The
initial experience was most encouraging. The subsequent eight years
have witnessed the birth of a revolution in medical practice.

The basic principle of the Coronary Care Unit at the time of its
inception was to place all patients with acute myocardial infarction
(AMI) in one area of the hospital. In this area there would be experienced nurses and physicians expert in resuscitation, and all patients

would be attached to an electrocardiographic monitor. The monitor alarms were set, and the staff then waited for the alarms to ring or for a cardiac arrest to develop. They then proceeded to resuscitate the patient. Over the years this concept of resuscitation has been useful and has resulted in a definite reduction in mortality. As experience developed, it became apparent that a different attitude toward the patients would result in a greater saving of lives. This attitude developed from the constant observation of the ECG minotor by the human eye to detect the very earliest arrhythmias (the early warning signs of impending disaster). (See Chap. 5 on Arrhythmia.) Subsequently the CCU was designed so that a knowledgeable person was present to observe the ECG monitor continuously for arrhythmia. The essence of the CCU shifted away from cardiac arrest to the detection of the early warning signs and prevention of life-threatening arrhythmia. This is the present status.

DETECTION AND TREATMENT OF "LIFE-THREATENING ARRHYTHMIA"

The essential features of the CCU are:
1. all patients with AMI are in one area of the hospital;
2. all the patients have continuous ECG monitoring;
3. a responsible, trained person observes the ECG continuously; and
4. the attitude of the staff is one of "aggressive management of cardiac arrhythmia."

It is apparent that the above can be carried out in practically any hospital. It can be done outside the hospital—i.e., in an ambulance, in stores, or at home (the Mobile Coronary Care Unit).

At first the ECG monitoring of the patient was done by a physician who was in continuous attendance at the monitor. This proved impractical over the years, as there were not enough physicians available and they were not temperamentally suited to sit at the monitor, hour after hour. The plan was then modified so that a nurse sat at the monitor bank and watched the oscilloscope to detect the arrhythmia. This, after trial, has likewise proven impractical because of the shortage of nurses and the need for their skills in other areas. Although many institutions continue to use nurses, there is a gradual shift to the use of paramedical personnel and technicians as monitor attendants (See Fig. 12).

Preparing for the Coronary Care Unit

Every hospital which admits patients with AMI should provide for the establishment of coronary care units, or send the patient to an institution where such a unit exists. Twenty-five admissions per year of patients with AMI should constitute the need for a separate Coronary Care Unit.

THE CCU COMMITTEE (OR MEDICAL-SURGICAL-NURSING PRACTICES COMMITTEE)

Each hospital should establish a committee to evaluate its own needs. However, continuous electrocardiographic monitoring of the acutely ill is here to stay. It is hardly conceivable that a hospital or community cannot afford a few thousand dollars for ECG monitors—the hardware. However, the software, or nursing staff, is another matter. Because of nursing staff problems it may not be possible for every hospital to have a CCU. Although it is felt that the larger hospitals can manage a unit more readily than the smaller ones, such is often not the truth, for there are many effective units functioning in small hospitals. In any community it is likely that very small hospitals would prefer to pool the resources of their area, rather than try to acquire individually the necessary staff that may not be efficiently utilized. In some rural areas such a plan is applicable. The community needs would be better serviced by a "regional" mobile coronary care team which would transport patients to a hospital with a fully equipped CCU, rather than have a unit in every hospital. Thus by pooling resources a community may better serve itself and its population.

Any hospital planning committee should consist of physicians, nurses, administrators, architects, electricians, and record librarians. Often, visits to established units save much planning time for all concerned. Also, there are many courses given across the country for nurses who are interested in CCU, and it cannot be stressed too strongly that the nurses run the unit. Their advice should be sought early in the planning stage.

PHYSICAL DESIGN

Once the essential goals of coronary care are appreciated, almost any hospital facility can be adapted. The following suggestions may be helpful. Although it has been stated that the ideal CCU is a separate unit with its own staff and chief, other systems are workable. Some continue to have the CCU as part of an Intensive Care Unit (ICU). Some have patients attached to monitors in various rooms on a floor. All over the country, and at innumerable meetings, one hears the following ideas expressed:

1. The CCU should be separate from the ICU (we feel that patients should be separated, although the units might be adjacent; Fig. 1).
2. Each patient should be in a separate room. There is no evidence on this point, and although many patients prefer separate rooms, not all do.
3. The unit should be in a part of the hospital where traffic of medical personnel is greatest. Presumably this insures ready availability of physicians for emergencies. The authors feel that this is overemphasized.,
4. The essence of the CCU is continuous electrocardiography and trained observation, not resuscitation.
5. The unit should be adjacent to the emergency room.
6. The unit should be adjacent to the post-anesthesia recovery room (PAR).
7. The surroundings should be cheerful and tranquil. This is emphasized so that the CCU patients are *not mixed* with patients recovering from anesthesia (PAR), those with serious trauma (ICU), or noisy and physically unmanageable patients (maximum security).

It is best to be guided by the "essential features" (page 000), apply them as best as practicable, and be guided by medical and not by architectural needs. As an extreme example, we are working on a plan to place ECG monitors a considerable distance from the patients and in another building. This is being considered because of the availability of technicians in the "other" building. They will also be watching the monitors of patients with illnesses other than AMI.

SIZE OF UNIT

The following, although from excellent sources, must be tempered by the guidelines already discussed. According to the National Conference on Coronary Care Units, the following formula may be applied to determine the bed capacity and is based on a statistical review of the number of discharged patients with AMI.

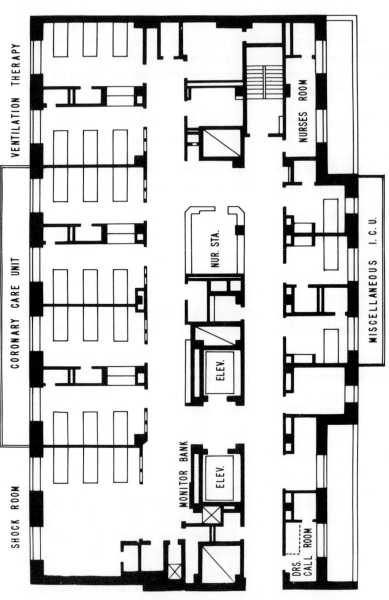

Fig. 1. Floor plan of the Coronary Care Unit at St. Vincent's Hospital. The CCU is physically separate from the ICU. A room is set aside for patients in shock or pulmonary edema. A doctor's "on call" room is present in the unit. A central monitor bank is located strategically away from the traffic at the nurses station. Private rooms are provided for security purposes and isolation. A separate assistant head nurse is ~~available for each of the major units. Shock, Coronary Care, and Ventilation (intensive respiratory~~

22

$$\text{Number of beds} = \frac{\text{Number of AMI per year} \times \text{Days in Unit}}{365}$$

It should be understood when deriving this formula that only about half of all patients admitted to a unit for suspected infarction actually prove to have a documented infarct.

Each bed should have a minimum of 130 to 150 square feet of floor space to allow for ample uncluttered working space. Each room should be under the direct vision of the nurses. Additional space should be set aside for the storage of equipment. A sleeping room and lounge for the physician on duty must be provided.

SPECIAL CONSIDERATIONS

1. Since the essence of the CCU is cardiac monitoring, the *electric circuitry* of the unit must be separate from that of the general hospital. Each electric outlet in the unit must have a common electric ground. The electric accidents reported in earlier years were almost all due to grounding problems which allowed electricity to leak from one machine to another and through the patient who was burned or shocked with AC current. Consultation with an electrical engineer must be made before any construction is contemplated. Four electric outlets per bed is the minimum. (ECG machine, extra light, cardiac monitor and defibrillator are frequently used almost simultaneously.)

2. Emergency electric power sources must be provided in case the usual power source fails. This should also provide emergency lighting, heat, and air-conditioning.

3. Central monitoring consoles (Fig. 2) are very useful in that they provide instant and continuous observation of cardiac rhythm of all patients. If less than four patients are monitored, "central consoles" are probably not necessary (Fig. 3).

4. Closed circuit television is feasible and may be employed in areas where direct observation of patients by the nurse is difficult (see Fig. 4).

5. Each bed should be provided with its own oxygen outlet, suction equipment, overhead light, and intravenous stand.

6. A hospital alarm system should be provided which can be activated by pushing a convenient button rather than dialing the telephone; the hospital operator, without further information, immediately announces over the page system that an emergency exists in the CCU (Fig. 5). A code system is preferred to minimize the concern which other patients experience when "cardiac arrest" is announced. St. Vincent's Hospital has adopted "Code 99" as a general announce-

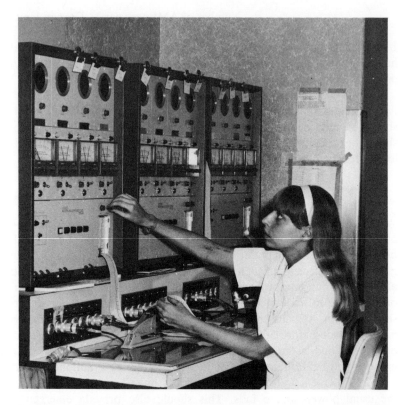

Fig. 2. Central Monitor Bank staffed by a technician. Each cardiac monitor is a duplicate of one outside the patient's room. An ECG readout is provided. Rhythm strips are recorded every hour by the technician and reviewed by a staff physician. Abrupt changes in cardiac rate or rhythm are immediately brought to the attention of the staff physician.

ment of a cardiac arrest. Other institutions use "Code Blue" or "Doctor Blue," and so on. A large wall-mounted clock or stopwatch, activated by pushing a button, is used in some institutions for timing a resuscitation.

7. A readily available volume-cycled respirator should be part of the equipment (Fig. 6).

8. Where possible the hospital should have a special room, more thoroughly outfitted with monitoring devices for patients in shock or congestive heart failure. This room may have an image intensifier for the insertion of pacemakers, a console for the direct measurement of

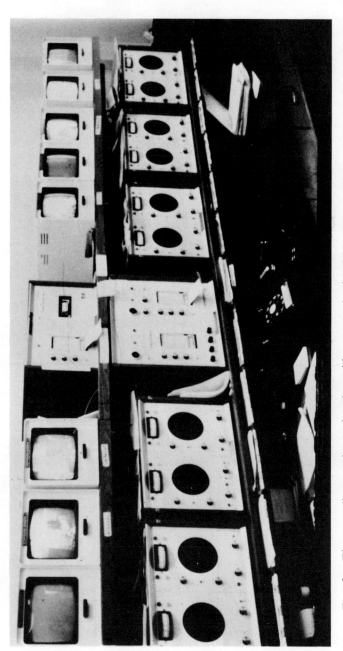

Fig. 3. Three cardiac monitors placed outside a room in the CCU. The monitors are easily seen by the nurse but away from the view of the patients. The photograph shows the essence of the hardware of coronary care; all the patients with suspected myocardial infarction are in one area and have continuous electrocardiographic monitoring.

25

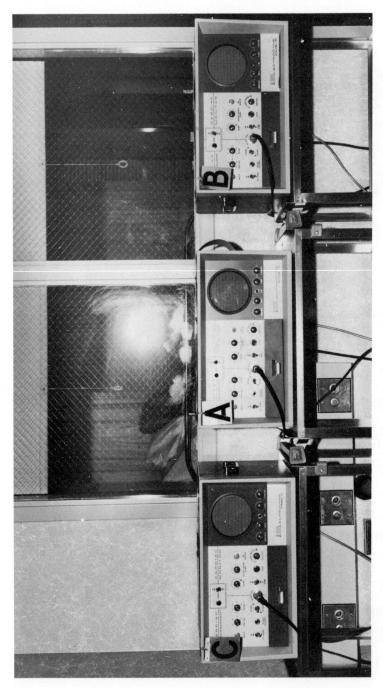

Fig. 4. Central Monitor Bank with closed circuit television. Such systems are feasible when patients are not visible at the nurse's station or when the quantity of nurses is insufficient to provide continuous bed-side attendance. (Courtesy of Mennon Gaetback Co.)

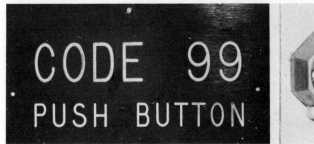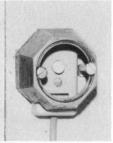

Fig. 5. A button in the wall which activates an alarm in the telephone room. The telephone operator without further information announces the emergency call for help in the CCU. At St. Vincent's Hospital this summons is called *"Code 99"*.

central aortic and central venous pressures, and a respirator for the treatment of inappropriate ventilation and hypoxemia. Ideally this room should be near the CCU. It is not mandatory to have such a room or to have it near the CCU. However, patients in shock or acute pulmonary edema should be moved away from the eyes of patients who are less acutely ill in the CCU. A catheterization laboratory is frequently used for the purpose of insertion of pacemakers; other institutions use a procedure room in the X-ray Department.

One of the fallacies which has grown up concerning the CCU is that establishment of a unit requires a staggering financial outlay with architectural changes and the acquisition of numerous pieces of electronic equipment. This contains an element of truth, but it is surprising how little is absolutely required to maintain a well-functioning unit. The following is a list of necessary equipment.

THE MONITOR

The ECG monitor is the *sine qua non* of coronary care. There are many models with varying degrees of sophistication produced by several electronic manufacturers. The essential features of any model should include the following (Fig. 7):

1. A screen which is easily visible. Minimum acceptability is a 5-inch screen with good tonal relief so that the heart rhythm can be detected at a distance. Some screens are green, others brown. The

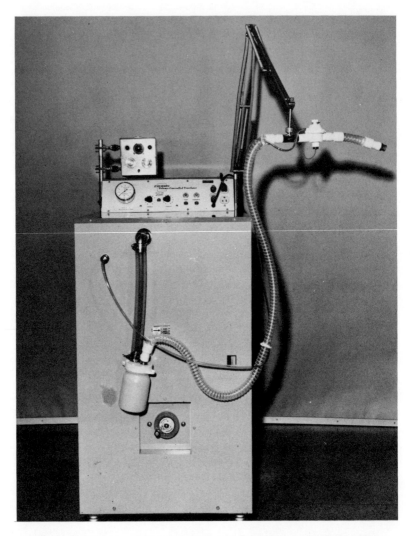

Fig. 6. A volume cycled respirator. In addition to standard parts, an apnea alarm is included which is activated by separation of the machine from an endotracheal tube or by malfunction of the machine.

color is not important. Newly manufactured equipment using predominantly solid state or transistorized circuits is far more steady and probably more durable than the original vacuum tube equipment.

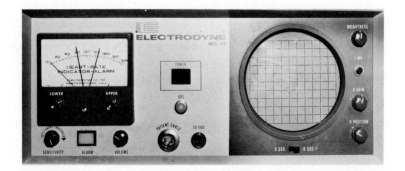

Fig. 7. Cardiac monitor with oscilloscope, heart rate meter and alarm. The ECG may be centered or modified in size by the V position and V gain, respectively. Limits of heart rate are selected and if exceded an adjustable alarm is activated. The sweep of the oscilloscope is changed from 3 to 6 seconds to identify ECG complexes.

2. The pulse rate meter is an essential adjunct to the monitor. An audible "beep" with each QRS is part of every machine. Fortunately the volume can be turned off or lowered, as it is impractical to have four to six "beepers" going simultaneously.

3. Alarms which can be set to ring at "high" and "low" cardiac rates are probably also essential. More recent equipment produces different tones for "high" and "low" frequency "alarms." This is not a critical requirement.

4. Durability: Most of the available equipment is remarkably rugged.

5. Service: This is most important. Avoid purchasing equipment that must be shipped out to be repaired. Local engineering firms, universities, or trade schools should be able to provide all repairs.

6. Memory unit: Instruments that will write out an ECG as a continuous record for the last 30 or 60 seconds preceding an arrhythmia are remarkable engineering accomplishments. Their practicability, in view of the expense, has not been clearly shown. They are not part of our equipment.

7. Multiple ECG leads: The ability to record from the patient all six leads ("frontal" plane) is an advantage, but it requires that the patient wear four electrodes. We feel that two electrodes are enough for an ECG lead and enough of a nuisance to the patient. If an arrhythmia occurs, the routine ECG machine should be used and a

12-lead cardiogram taken so that the proper interpretation of the arrhythmia may be made.

THE PATIENT ELECTRODES

THE ELECTRODE

The patient is attached to the monitor by wires. The end of the wire on the patient's chest may be a small subcutaneous needle, or any one of a large variety of salt suspension silver electrodes. We prefer the needle electrodes because they require little attention once they are placed. They actually cause very little discomfort and they stay in place. This is of paramount importance in saving time when one is monitoring 8 to 12 patients at the same time. When there are only two to four patients, the time-saving aspect of the needles is of less importance. The needles are of conducting metal, 26-gauge, 1 inch in length, and disposable. They are secured with paper adhesive tape and are changed every 2 to 3 days. The lead cables are secured to the abdomen with paper tape, so that traction on the cable will not dislodge the electrode needles.

There are many varieties of electrodes available; there is no substantiated experience to say that one is better than another. More important is the care with which they are applied. Any of the small silver plate types will work well if carefully applied. In over 1,000 patients we have had only a few minor infections. A local ecchymotic area around the needle is usually all that results from their use.

LOCATION

Ideally, the electrodes should be placed so that the line between them overlies and is parallel to the mean QRS vector. This will produce the tallest R wave and, in general, is the most satisfactory lead. This vector is generally parallel to the Lead II axis of the frontal plane ECG (right arm to left leg). The electrode on the patient's left is positive, that on his right is negative.

For practical purposes, one electrode (negative) is placed on the right side of the patient's chest, and the other (positive) on the left side slightly inferior to that on the right side. Both are roughly on the level of the 4th and 5th interspace, lateral to the mid-clavicular lines. We place the needles in the anterior axillary fold where the skin is soft. Needles cannot be placed over the ribs because the tightness of the skin makes them uncomfortable. The silver electrodes which are applied to the chest wall with adhesive tape may be placed as follows: one in the 2nd right interspace at the sternal edge; the other in the 4th interspace in the mid-clavicular line. If the R wave is small, compare it with the ECG Leads I, II, and III. Adjust the placement of the electrodes so that the line between the electrodes is parallel to the ECG vector showing the tallest R wave (Fig. 8).

Lead   I: right to left across the chest, at the same level.

Lead II: right to left, vertically across the heart, right higher than left.

Lead III: left to right across the chest, right more inferior than left.

FALSE ALARMS

Two types of false alarm occur: a) low frequency, or "asystole," and b) high frequency false alarms. The most common condition associated with "asystole" false alarm is the attendant forgetting to notify the monitor personnel that the electrodes were being removed. Generally this is due to carelessness and can be avoided by meticulous attention to details of electrode placement, and by communication between various persons in the unit. Other reasons include dislodgement of the needles, broken wires, and decrease in the voltage

ELECTRODE   PLACEMENT

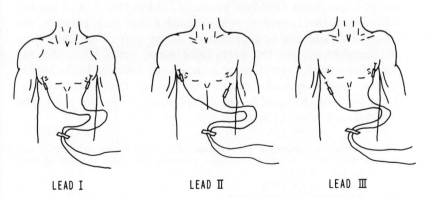

LEAD I   LEAD II   LEAD III

Fig. 8.   The electrode lead position demonstrated approximates the ECG leads as indicated.

"gain" of the monitor. Low frequency false alarms are unusual and must be investigated by going to the bedside. High frequency false alarms are due to the electrodes detecting electric energy associated with muscle contraction when the patient moves, or with the sustained muscle contraction of heavy breathing or muscle tension. The electrodes pick up this electric energy and the electric circuits of the monitor "count" it as pulse and register it on the rate meter, which jumps suddenly to 250-300. Characteristically, it appears as "static" on the oscilloscope screen. Experienced persons can generally recognize this, but it is not always easy. There is as yet no satisfactory system of eliminating this type of false alarm without eliminating the QRS itself in its proper form and rate.

THE DEFIBRILLATOR

The electric defibrillator is the single most important therapeutic tool in the Coronary Care Unit. Every unit should have two such instruments, for, although generally sturdy and reliable, they occasionally break down. Several models are available. Common to all are the following (Fig. 9):

1. A source of variable energy measured in watt-seconds.* The AC defibrillator was used extensively in earlier years because of the work of Kouwenhoven during the 1930's. The limitations of the AC defibrillator were well known. It sometimes induced ventricular fibrillation. The dose could not be programmed accurately and the heat generated was enormous. The superiority of the DC defibrillator became abundantly clear when it was introduced by Lown. The energy requirement (and heat produced) is less than that of the AC defibrillator, the current is unidirectional rather than pulsatile, the energy discharge can be programmed to any part of the QRS cycle and, empirically, the DC defibrillator often works when the AC defibrillator fails. The difference in the energy delivered to the patient is more readily appreciated when one realizes that 6,000 volts $\times$ 0.001 second is delivered by DC defibrillation, as opposed to 60 volts $\times$ 0.1 second delivered by AC.

---

* When a unit is capable of programming the time of dose delivery at any point in the QRS, it is called a cardioverter. Most units have a range of from one to 400 watt seconds.

    Watt = volts $\times$ amps

    Watt seconds = watt $\times$ time

Some defibrillators express the variable energy source as Joules, which is the same as watt seconds $\times$ heat coefficient.

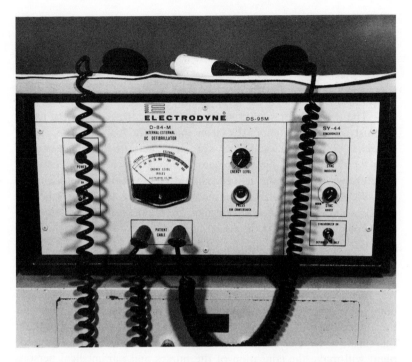

Fig. 9. DC defibrillator. A variable source of energy is selected by a dial and the amount displayed on a meter. A button on the console is provided to discharge the machine. The paddles are always plugged in and stored neatly on the machine. Electrode paste is readily available. Note the switch in the lower right corner which converts the defibrillator to a cardioverter. See text for details.

2. Conducting plates or paddles: These paddles must be easily maneuverable and easily placed on the chest wall. Paddles which require elaborate placement on the posterior thorax are unacceptable for a defibrillator because there is not one second to waste. The paddles must be kept meticulously clean.

3. A depolarizing switch or button protected against accidental discharge. Discharge buttons on the paddles are sometimes hazardous. Discharge buttons on the defibrillator console, while they require an additional hand, are probably safer, and the operator can pay full attention to the proper placement of the paddles. Premature discharge of the electric current may shock the patient, or the operator, and may produce a severe burn of the patient's chest. Depolarizing switches triggered by foot pedals are less acceptable because of fre-

quent accidental discharges and the time required to set them up. If only one person is on duty, the activating button must be on the paddle. Otherwise we prefer the activating button on the body of the instrument.

4. An adapter switch so that the machine can be switched from defibrillator to cardioverter in an instant.

The defibrillator should be located in a central area of the CCU. It must be kept meticulously clean and ready for use. The paddle wires are "plugged in" and ready for use. Electrode jelly must be kept with the defibrillator. No other paraphernalia which may conceivably interfere with its prompt delivery should be stored with the defibrillator. No cover is placed on the machine. The electric cord (the AC cord) is loosely placed so that it may be removed quickly. The technique of defibrillation is discussed in another section, under "Arrhythmias" (p. 87).

STANDARDIZATION OF EQUIPMENT

All electronic instruments should be acquired from the same company. This will insure the substitution of one part for another and the interchange of one instrument for another. It is imperative that the cardioverter can be used with the monitor. Uniformity of equipment will make the education of the nurses and paramedical personnel less difficult.

THE RESUSCITATION CART
(the "Crash" cart or "Code" cart)

The "crash" cart is a suitable cart, not top-heavy, readily movable, on large wheels, and stocked with various items (Fig. 10). The equipment kept on our cart is itemized in Table 1. Of importance is the open display of needles and syringes, so that they are readily found in the called-for size.

TABLE 1. *Resuscitation Cart Inventory*

TOP SHELF:

1. Cabinet with Medications (ampule files taped on side)
2. Package containing:
   a) laryngoscope with blade
   b) endotracheal tube with stylet
   c) clamp and syringe
3. Ambu Bag with Face Mask
4. Assorted Endotracheal Tubes (#20, 32, 34, 36, 38, 40)
5. Clamps with Rubber Tips

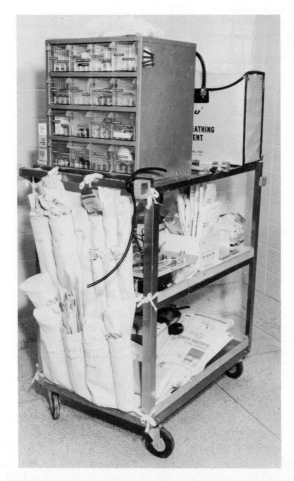

Fig. 10. The "crash cart." A mobile cart stocked with accessible medicine and equipment. Ampoules of medicine are labelled and placed in transparent containers. An ample supply of syringes and needles of various sizes is available. The various packets facilitate the finding of the proper size of needle or syringe. Equipment is neatly placed on open shelves. An inventory is listed elsewhere.

SECOND SHELF:

1. Veno Packs (Macro/Micro Drips)
2. Blood Transfusion Sets
3. Veno Caths (#14-18)
4. I.V. Solutions (Isotonic Salines, 5% D/S, 5% D/W and Sodium Bicarbonate)

5. Merthiolate
6. 4 x 4, 2 x 2 adhesive tape and Lubafax
7. Levine Tubes—Endotracheal Tube Cuffs
8. Endotracheal Tray with Bite Block
9. Assorted Adapters

BOTTOM SHELF:

1. Cutdown Set
2. Scalpel
3. Sterile Gloves

4. Irrigating Set
5. Blood Pump*

BAG ON SIDE OF CART:

1. 20 cc Syringes
2. 10 cc Syringes
3. 2 cc Syringes

4. Intra-cardiac Needles
5. Needles (#15, 18, 20, 22, 25)
6. Tourniquets

CODE CART MEDICATIONS:

1. Epinephrine
2. Aminophylline
3. Atropine
4. Aramine
5. Benadryl
6. Calcium Chloride
7. Calcium Gluconate
8. Cedilanid
9. Digoxin
10. Dextrose 50%
11. Isuprel
12. Morphine Sulfate

13. Neosynephrine
14. Ouabain
15. Potassium Chloride
16. Xylocaine
17. Pronestyl
18. Quinidine
19. Ethacrynic Acid
20. Furosemide
21. Tubocurarine
22. Na Bicarbonate
23. Solu-Cortef
24. Bretyllium

A PORTABLE ELECTROCARDIOGRAPH

This machine should be the sole property of the CCU and immediately available to record changes in rhythm and to record daily standard electrocardiograms. All personnel on the CCU should know how to position and apply the electrodes. Two chest cups should be available for doing the "Lewis" lead. An esophageal lead must be available.

A BATTERY-POWERED PACEMAKER

At least two "demand"-type pacemakers are required, with a good supply of catheter pacemakers.

---

* The cuff to put around blood container.

THE MECHANICAL CHEST COMPRESSOR

A mechanical chest compressor is a useful device during cardiac resuscitation. It is probably more effective than the arms of the physician or nurse, and it is certainly less tiring. Many such devices are available. They vary from complex "heart lung" resuscitators to simple machine compressors. Some are driven by compressed O_2, and some are electrically driven. The complex chest compressor and pulmonary ventilator are very effective when properly applied and supervised. They require a great deal of experience to keep them in working order and are probably best used by large hospitals. Small units, not requiring frequent use, are best equipped with simple mechanical systems (Fig. 11).

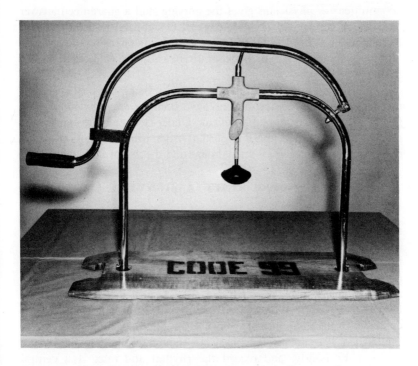

Fig. 11. A mechanical device used for closed-chest cardiac massage. The wooden board is placed under the patient and the aluminum bar inserted into sprockets. An adjustable rubber piston is provided. Cardiac massage may be carried out for long periods of time without fatigue.

Staffing the
Coronary Care Unit

ATTENDING PHYSICIANS

Many staffing patterns are adaptable and many variations are in operation throughout the country.

1. Attending physician: full time, having no other major responsibility. He may be physically present or in an adjacent office all the time.

2. Resident, or intern physician, physically present at all times.

3. One or more attending physicians, each spending a few hours a day in the unit and, when not present, immediately available by telephone. This combination of emergency "hot line" telephone and a "committee" of physicians gives the nursing staff a guaranteed answer to a telephone call 24 hours a day. ECG's can be transmitted over telephone lines to the doctor's office by the persons using this system.

4. Nurse in charge, backed up by a physician available by phone.

Ideally a physician covers the CCU by being physically present at all times. Very few institutions have such coverage available, and for a small unit it is not practical. Under such circumstances the nurses will play their most important roles after instruction in the diagnosis and treatment of arrhythmias and the use of the defibrillator.

HOUSE STAFF ASSIGNMENT IN THE CCU

The house staff physician will examine every patient immediately upon admission to the CCU, take a careful history, and institute whatever immediate therapy is necessary. He will take, or examine, a full 12-lead electrocardiogram. He should then notify the referring physician and advise him of the patient's condition. Each day the resident or intern will make rounds on every patient in the unit with the Unit Director or his representative. Differences of opinion will be discussed with the attending physician and a plan of action for that day established. The house staff physician should see the patient, inspect the monitor hourly, and record the rhythm and rate. If a central console is present, the resident should review "rhythm" strips hourly and record abnormalities on the chart. Whenever arrhythmias are present he should obtain arterial blood for gas analysis. He is the physician-in-charge of resuscitation unless a more senior ranking physician is present at the time of a cardiac arrest and wishes to take charge.

The essence of success is availability. The house officer should never leave the unit unless relieved by another physician of equal competence. At first, only resident physicians are assigned to the unit. As the academic year progresses and the interns become more familiar with hospital routine and policy, they are selectively assigned to the unit, depending on their degree of competence.

NURSING STAFF

There should be at least one registered nurse on duty at all times. She should be assisted by practical nurses and nurses' aides. Highly motivated and trained women can be of exceptional service by relieving the nurse of lesser responsibilities, such as making beds, recording temperatures and so on, and by assisting her in providing better medical care to the patient. The nurse should be selected for continuing education by the medical staff so that there will always be a nurse on duty who can translate the monitor rhythm to her staff and make sound decisions before calling the doctor or initiating therapy. How many patients a nurse can care for depends upon how much of her time is taken up with non-nursing duties and how much assistance she has. Nursing responsibilities are given in more detail in the section, "Nursing Aspects of the CCU" (Chapter 9).

UNIT SECRETARY (MANAGER)

It should be the responsibility of one person to direct traffic in the unit. Non-medical personnel can fill this role satisfactorily. The secretary keeps track of admissions, transfers, and discharges and limits visitors to whatever standard is set by the hospital. She may be responsible for inventory of machinery. She answers the telephone and places calls for the nurses and doctors in the unit. Other secretarial chores may be assigned, depending on local custom and practice.

OXYGEN THERAPIST

It is difficult for even a large CCU to command the use of a full-time oxygen therapist. Most hospitals have a local pool of oxygen therapists who administer treatment throughout the hospital. It is advantageous to select one or two therapists to discharge most of their responsibilities in the CCU, so that the same people become familiar with the special needs and treatments which only infrequently are required outside the unit. In this way, certain paramedical personnel become part of the team and participate in the daily practice.

ELECTRONIC TECHNICIANS

In units where there is a large collection of electronic equipment, it may be necessary to have a person who is familiar with electronics oversee and keep in repair the myriad electric equipment that is flooding the CCU. Most electronic failures are due to simple problems—worn batteries, tubes, broken wires, and blown fuses. It requires someone with a special interest to look after these machines and see that they are always in proper working order. This is not the nurse's job (Fig. 12).

PARAMEDICAL PERSONNEL

The list of people with specialized knowledge is endless. There are dieticians, social workers, psychologists, clergy and housekeepers. Nothing is special about the service which these people provide in the CCU that differs from that in the general hospital. By nature, most people who work in a hospital want to participate in patient care. In setting up a CCU, it is a long-term investment to seek early the council of all paramedical personnel involved. The sheer force of their enthusiasm and desire to participate will make the burden of running a unit less onerous.

We have a special interest in using ECG technicians to operate the monitor bank (Fig. 2).

TABLE 2. *Minimum Equipment for CCU*

Electronic monitor	one per patient
(5″ scope + rate meter and alarm)	one in reserve
Electric D.C. defibrillator—cardioverter	2 per CCU
ECG machine	one for the unit
	standby in general hospital
O_2	one source of O_2 per bed
Suction	one source per bed
Mechanical respirator	one in CCU
	standby in general hospital
Crash cart	one in CCU
Mechanical chest compressor	one in CCU per unit

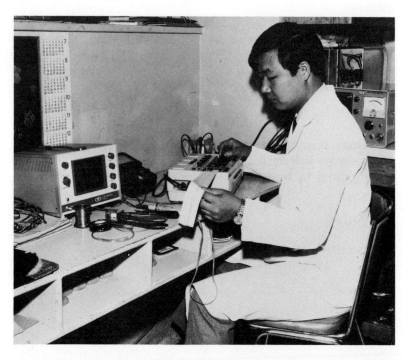

Fig. 12. An electronic engineer at his workbench. He must be familiar with the wiring diagrams of all the equipment and be able to make repairs. Thus long delays for repairs are eliminated. An electronic technician to make minor repairs, i.e., of cables and tubes, would also be of great help.

POLICIES IN MOST CCU'S

VISITORS:

All patients admitted with a diagnosis of acute myocardial infarction are necessarily placed on the critical list. It is only natural for friends and family to want to visit the critically ill patient. In order to avoid the horde of visitors who descend on the unit, a limit is placed on their number. Only two visitors per patient for 5 minutes of the hour are allowed. The most responsible member of the family decides who the visitors may be. This policy is well accepted by the family in most cases. The unit secretary keeps track of the traffic.

SMOKING:

Smoking is forbidden in the CCU for all patients. Members of the staff who desire to smoke must do so in their lounge or off the unit.

RADIOS:

Small personal transistor radios with ear listening pieces are acceptable if patients desire them. We know of no problems with electric energy release from these small radios.

TELEVISION:

No television is permitted in the CCU.

FLOWERS:

General hospital policy is followed.

TELEPHONES:

None are permitted to patients.

References

Balagot, R. C., and Bandelin, U. R. Comparative evaluation of some D.C. cardiac defibrillators. Amer. Heart J., 77:489, 1969.

Beck, C. S., Weckhesser, F. C., and Barry, F. M. Fatal heart attack and surgical defibrillation. J.A.M.A., 161:434, 1956.

Church, G., and Biern, R. O. Intensive coronary care. System for a small hospital without house staff. New Eng. J. Med., 281:1155, 1969.

Day, H. W. An intensive coronary care area. Dis. Chest, 44:432, 1963.

Decker, D. D. Coronary Care Units Without House Staffs. Presented at regional meeting of A.C.C.P., Halsted, Kansas. Hertzler Clinic, Sept. 21, 1969.

Frommer, P. L. The myocardial infarction research program of the National Heart Institute. Amer. J. Cardiol., 22:108, 1968.

Grace, W. J. The use of paramedical personnel in the coronary care unit. Clin. Res. XVII, 4:616, 1969.

———— and Soscia, J. L. Reducing mortality from acute myocardial infarction—current ideas. Cardiol. Digest, 4:29, 1969.

———— and Minogue, W. F. Electrocardiographic monitoring services: a technical point. Amer. J. Cardiol., 16:300, 1965.

Guidelines for Coronary Care Units. U.S. Dept. of Health, Education and Welfare, July, 1968. Public Health Service Publications No. 1824.

Jude, J. R., and Elam, J. O. Fundamentals of Cardiopulmonary Resuscitation. Philadelphia, F. A. Davis Company, 1965.

Lown, B., Fakhro, A. M., Hood, W. B., Jr., and Thorn, G. W. The coronary unit, J.A.M.A., 199:188, 1967.

Marshall, R. M., and Bloun, S. G., Jr., Acute myocardial infarction —influence of a coronary care unit. Arch. Int. Med., 122:472, 1968.

Oliver, M. F., Julian, D. G., and Donald, K. W. Problems in evaluating coronary care units. Their responsibilities and their relation to the community. Amer. J. Cardiol., 20:465, 1967.

Pearson, J. W. Historical and Experimental Approaches to Modern Resuscitation. Springfield, Ill., Charles C Thomas, Publisher, 1965.

Proceedings of the Conference on Impact of a Coronary Care Unit, on Hospital, Medical Practice and Community. Arlington, Virginia, Heart Disease Control Program National Center for Chronic Disease Control, 1966.

Proceedings of the National Conference on Coronary Care Units. U.S. Dept. of Health, Education and Welfare, March, 1968, Public Health Publication No. 1764.

Shaw, G., Smith, G., and Thompson, F. A. Resuscitation and Cardiac Pacing. Philadelphia, F. A. Davis Company, 1965.

Shillingford, J. P., and Thomas, M. The organization of a unit for the intensive care and investigation of patients with acute myocardial infarction. Lancet, 2:1113, 1964.

Smith, W. G. A coronary care unit in a general medical ward. Lancet, 2:397, 1968.

Surwaciz, B., and Pellegrino, E. D. Sudden Cardiac Death. New York, Grune & Stratton, Inc., 1964.

Wyman, M., and Hammersmith, L. Coronary care in the small community hospital. Dis. Chest, 53:584, 1968.

Yu, P. N., Imboden, C. A., Fox, S. M., and Killip, T. Coronary care unit (1) and (2). Mod. Conc. Cardiovasc. Dis., 34:23, 1965.

3

General Therapy of
Acute Myocardial Infarction

The treatment of myocardial infarction includes both modern and traditional procedures. Although more emphasis is placed on modern treatments, which have been developed in the past decade, the traditional features of treatment will not be overlooked. Traditionally, the treatment of myocardial infarction includes the prescription of bed rest, diet, sedation and the like, treatment which is common to many illnesses. These stereotyped treatments, however, have been critically reappraised in the light of a better understanding of physiology, and rigid prescription is no longer the rule.

Modern treatment of myocardial infarction is accepted, not so much because it is new, but because it saves lives. The ability to treat life-threatening arrhythmia has led to the development of a regimen for myocardial infarction not imagined just a decade ago. The isolated patient in a darkened room with a private nurse has been replaced by a community of sick patients electronically monitored, provided with sophisticated drugs and electronic devices. While the individuality of patient care is seemingly lessened, the patient now has a better chance of leaving the hospital alive. The following is a description of the combination of traditional and modern treatment of acute myocardial infarction as it is employed today. Hopefully, what we consider modern will soon be traditional.

Bed Rest

Bed rest continues to be the basis of treatment, but its duration and degree have changed radically in recent years. The usual prescription was for 6 weeks of total bed rest based on evidence that it took 2 to 3 weeks for collateral circulation to appear and 6 weeks for fibrosis to be complete in the infarcted myocardium. Present guidelines consist of a 3-week total hospitalization for the patient with an uncomplicated myocardial infarction. The patient is admitted to the Coronary Care Unit, where bed rest is enforced for from 5 to 7 days. Initially, he is not permitted to feed or wash himself. A bedside commode may be used if the blood pressure is stable. The recumbent position is preferable during the first few days, but if the blood pressure is normal, the patient may be in a semi-recumbent position several hours a day, or up in a chair for a few hours. During the second week, he may sit in a chair for several hours a day in divided time until he can sit up continuously without fatigue. During the second week he may take a few steps in his room. In the third week, ambulation may be increased so that the patient may walk freely, but slowly, in the corridors of the hospital. If the patient's illness is complicated by congestive heart failure, shock, or pulmonary embolus, ambulation as described above is estimated from the time of the disappearance of the complication.

The armchair treatment, although theoretically more advantageous in terms of diminishing cardiac demands, is impractical in the modern hospital. So few patients die of pulmonary embolus that it is difficult to build a strong case for the chair treatment. In every case, ambulation should be individualized to the patient's needs. We have rarely found it necessary to hospitalize a patient for more than one month. We have outlined a series of instructions for the house staff as follows:

Management of Patients with Myocardial Infarction

The patient with myocardial infarction will be managed according to the following regimen. Advanced age, debilitation and/or complications may modify the regimen.

HOSPITAL DAY	LOCATION	GENERAL MANAGEMENT
1st to 7th Hospital Day	CCU	All patients have O_2 and I.V. On critical. Continuous monitor; coronary precautions.* Heparin is routine. 1,600 calorie diet, regular.
Beginning 2nd Day:	CCU	O.O.B. ½ hour T.I.D. May use commode for B.M.
4th to 7th Hospital Day:	CCU	Self-feeding and shaving from day 4; D/C O_2, I.V. drip and coronary precautions.
7th or 8th Day: 7th or 8th Hospital Day to 11th Hospital Day	Transfer to ICCU	O.O.B. 1 hour T.I.D.+ and increase so that by 10 days patient is 6 hours O.O.B./day. EKG monitor strip every 4 hours. Attach adhesive electrode cables.
12th to 14th Day:	ICCU	B.R.P. Continue rhythm strip. Begin walking and gradually increase.
20th to 21st Hospital Day:	Discharge from ICCU	On 21st hospital day, up and about *ad lib*, to be discharged in a few days. *Check cardiac series.* Off critical.
Day of Discharge:		Anticoagulants continued up to day of discharge (21st day).
Entire Hospital Course:		1,600 calorie diet throughout hospital course.

* *By coronary precautions is meant:* Strict bed rest unless otherwise ordered. Patients should be assisted at meals—not necessarily fed. Patients should be shaved and bathed. Vital signs every four hours unless ordered more often. Patients may use transistor radio with earphone; may use light reading material.

Elastic Bandages for the Legs

In former years, when lengthy bed rest was prescribed, elastic bandages were often applied to the legs to enhance venous return. With earlier ambulation, we do not find this necessary. Phlebitis seems to be disappearing from the list of in-hospital complications.

The presence of varicose veins with stasis dermatitis warrants concern. The treatment then should include a pair of snugly fitting elastic stockings. Elastic bandages are discouraged because they more often act as tourniquets than aids to circulation.

Diet

The relationship of arteriosclerotic coronary artery disease and diet has been pointed out by Ancel Keys. The Framingham study a decade ago revealed a fourfold incidence of coronary artery disease in men with elevated serum cholesterol (above 225 mg percent) compared to a matched group with normal serum cholesterol. The Prudent Diet has been shown to effectively reduce the serum cholesterol level and presumably the incidence of coronary artery disease. A nutritious diet, easily digestible and free of gastric irritants (spices, sauces, etc.), should be prescribed for the patient with acute myocardial infarction. Our "routine" is a 1,600-calorie, low fat, low cholesterol, regular diet.

Low sodium diets are not required unless the patient is in overt congestive heart failure. Supplemental vitamins may be prescribed, but there is little evidence that they are of any value. Total caloric intake should not exceed 1,600 calories per day. During the first few days of hospitalization most patients have little appetite even for this limited amount of food. If it appears from the outset that the patient's condition is complicated and may require intubation or cardioversion, then a liquid diet may be desirable to decrease the likelihood of vomiting and the possibility of aspiration pneumonia. Four glasses of low sodium milk per day, the Karell Diet, are well tolerated.

Bowel Care

Bowel care is more than an incidental feature in the management of a patient with a life-threatening illness. Most analgesics are constipating and bed rest is not conducive to orderly bowel function. A bowel movement becomes the prime concern of some patients after several days of constipation. Unless the patient becomes quite distended, or uncomfortable, nothing needs to be done about the constipation for many days. A bedside commode is easier to use than a bed pan and may be used without danger at any time if the blood pressure is normal (Fig. 1). A bed pan should be avoided, for it frequently results in a vigorous Valsalva maneuver. This maneuver (more vigorously performed on the bed pan than a commode) reduces venous return to the heart, may reduce cardiac output and cause syncope, or the resulting increased venous pressure may strip off a blood clot in the legs. The "bed pan apoplexy" of former years is much less common now, but still occurs. To reduce straining at stool, a stool softener such as Colace, 100 mg twice a day, or Surfak, one tablet every day, is recommended. Sometimes, after several days of constipation, the use of one Dulcolax suppository will produce a bowel movement. If an enema seems necessary, it may be used without danger after the first few hospital days in most patients.

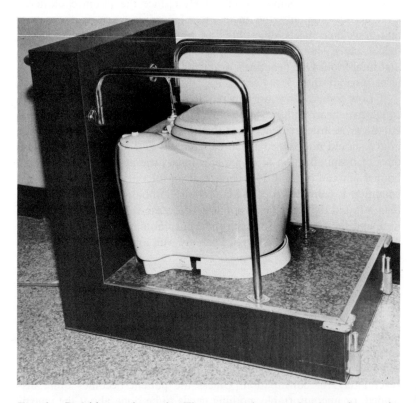

Fig. 1. Bedside septic tank. The commode may be brought to the patient's bedside and flushed without handling the contents.

Analgesics and Sedatives

Analgesic therapy should be individually tailored to the patient. This point cannot be overemphasized. Pain thresholds vary from one patient to another. Narcotics are too often prescribed by rote. After several hours in the hospital the patient is too often found stuporous with shallow respiration because of too liberal use of a narcotic. No more than two injections of a narcotic were required to relieve pain in over 300 patients with myocardial infarction at St. Vincent's Hospital. Excessive administration of analgesics, especially morphine, leads to hypoventilation and hypoxia.

For an average sized man, 10 mg of morphine sulfate may be administered intramuscularly as an initial dose. If pain continues after 20 minutes an additional dose may be required. Morphine has strong vagotropic properties which were not fully appreciated until recently. Morphine alone is associated with profound bradycardia and even cardiac arrest. For this reason, 0.4 mg atropine sulfate is always prescribed in conjunction with morphine for acute myocardial infarction. Formerly, atropine was prescribed to prevent vomiting but it now seems clear that the efficacy of atropine is related to vagolysis and the prevention of bradycardia, although the combination has not been investigated systematically. Demerol is an adequate substitute for morphine. An equivalent starting dose is 75 mg intramuscularly. The vagal effect of demerol is not as pronounced as morphine and it does not depress respiration as much. The administration of analgesics intravenously is rarely necessary. There is little evidence to support the belief that the intravenous route must be used in shock or that analgesia will itself relieve the shock state in myocardial infarction. Patients in cardiogenic shock do not, as a rule, complain of pain. Similarly, in congestive heart failure or in acute pulmonary edema, the intravenous administration of narcotics that suddenly depress the respiratory center may be hazardous. In every case, Nalline should be available to counteract any idiosyncrasy to these narcotic drugs.

Hypnotics and sedatives are not considered to be as important as they once were. The patient who suffers a heart attack is usually anxious. The anxiety of the patient, however, is often proportional to that of the physician. The reassurance of an even-tempered physician is all that most patients require. Based on data relating arrhythmia to alkalosis and hypoxemia, there is no reason to sedate the patient to the point where he is asleep most of the day and hypoventilating. Some patients will require sedation despite all efforts of reassurance. For this purpose Librium, 10 mg three times per day, or phenobarbitol, 30 mg three times per day, is satisfactory. Analgesics and hypnotics are a lethal combination during the first few days of myocardial infarction. The patient who is hypoxic from a damaged pump may be made further anoxic by having his respirations impaired.

Anticoagulants

No therapeutic modality has stirred more controversy than the use of anticoagulants in the treatment of acute myocardial infarction. Large series both for and against the use of anticoagulant therapy have been reported from every major nation in the world. No firm conclusions can yet be made. There is widespread agreement that anticoagulants have no effect on arrhythmias, shock or rupture of the ventricle. It is also accepted, even by the reports which show no reduction in mortality, that the incidence of thromboembolic phenemenon is significantly reduced. The recently popular practice of randomizing treatment on the basis of "good risk" and "poor risk" patients seems unjustified because the disease is so unpredictable. For the following reasons, all patients with acute myocardial infarction at St. Vincent's Hospital and Medical Center of New York are given anticoagulant therapy unless a specific contraindication is present:

1. Twenty-five percent of all patients who are admitted as Class I, or good risk, suffer a catastrophe, i.e., cardiac arrest.

2. Congestive heart failure is an insidious and often subclinical feature of myocardial infarction. There is a higher incidence of thromboembolism and pulmonary infarction in patients with congestive heart failure.

3. Hypoxemia is part and parcel of acute myocardial infarction. Studies at our hospital show that this is caused by venoarterial shunting of blood due to atelectasis and hypoventilation. Anticoagulants may have an effect in reducing the sludging of blood. While this is unproved, it merits serious consideration.

Anticoagulation is withheld from those patients who have a definite contraindication to the drug, e.g., previous bleeding peptic ulcer, subarachnoid hemorrhage, or known esophageal varices. The anticoagulant is discontinued in the presence of a pericardial friction rub, or in the face of complications of the drug itself, e.g., hematuria.

Warfarin, Coumadin and other drugs which interfere with pro-thrombin are no longer routinely used. At St. Vincent's Hospital, heparin sodium is the treatment of choice. A standard dose of 7,500 units every 6 hours is administered intravenously through an indwell-ing scalp vein needle inserted in the forearm or hand (Fig. 2). A Lee-White clotting time is performed one-half hour before the second dose. The dose is adjusted so that the clotting time is about twice

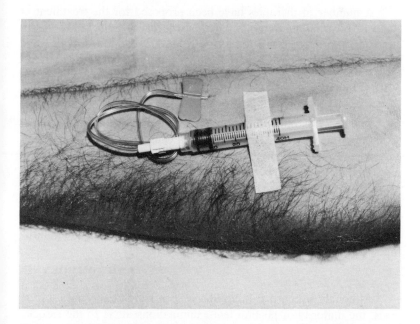

Fig. 2. Method of administering Heparin. A scalp vein needle is inserted intravenously and connected to a syringe. Heparin is administered period-ically by separating the plastic tubing from the syringe and injecting the dose. The remaining Heparin in the tubing and needle prevent clotting between injections. Adhesive tape has been eliminated for demonstration. This system may last for as long as the hospitalization but is usually changed weekly. This is called "the Heparin lock."

normal. Anticoagulation is carried on through the entire hospitalization. Some physicians discontinue the drug when the patient begins to walk. Intravenous heparin is administered by the nurse. The indwelling scalp vein needle eliminates the necessity of frequent subcutaneous or intramuscular heparin administration which often cause ecchymosis and pain. The scalp vein needle is well tolerated and no infections have resulted from its use. Rarely, a superficial chemical phlebitis occurs which disappears soon after the needle is removed.

Miscellaneous Therapies: Experimental, Abandoned

A number of therapies have been proposed for the treatment of acute myocardial infarction in the past decade. Some have merit, although unproved, while others have been abandoned with good reason. The following is a partial list of the more popular programs.

POLARIZING SOLUTIONS

Sodi-Pallares introduced this therapy based on the premise that arrhythmia in myocardial infarction was caused by potassium imbalance in the infarcted myocardium. Therapy consists of the intravenous administration of potassium salts, insulin, and dextrose solution in an attempt to repolarize the myocardial membranes. The initial enthusiasm for this procedure has not stood the test of time, and further studies have not confirmed a reduction in mortality. We have not observed any reduction in mortality or arrhythmias when the polarizing solution was used.

THROMBOLYSIN

Although myocardial infarction is seen without coronary thrombosis, the majority of postmortem examinations attest to the association of infarction and coronary thrombosis. Theoretically, lysis of the thrombus might alleviate the symptoms and even prevent infarction. To date, no thrombolytic substance has performed *in vivo* what has been expected of it on a theoretical basis. One report showed an improvement in the electrocardiogram, but no clinical improvement. The electrocardiographic changes appear to be a telescoping in time of the sequential changes normally seen. This form of therapy merits further study.

HYPERBARIC OXYGEN

Oxygen has been prescribed for decades with measurable improvement in blood pressure, peripheral resistance and oxygen tension. Based on this information and considering the difficulties in oxygenating some patients, investigations at one atmosphere hyperbaric oxygen were carried out in patients with acute myocardial infarction. A progressive rise in arterial pressure, peripheral resistance and oxygen tension, proceeding from one to two atmospheres of pressure, was noted. Concomitantly, there was a slight decrease in cardiac output and no effect on heart rate. If excess lactate was present before the use of hyperbaric oxygen, lactate was decreased. Hyperbaric oxygen may afford more than conventional therapy, but the size of the staff required, its limited availability and the cost of equipment relegate this procedure to the research center.

References

Burch, G. E., and Ansari, A. U. Bed rest, diet, nursing and environment. Amer. Heart J., 77:1, 1969.

Brown, K. W. G., and MacMillan, R. L. *In* Nichol, E. S., ed. Anticoagulant Therapy in Ischaemic Heart Disease. New York, Grune & Stratton, Inc., 1965, p. 70.

Cameron, A. J. V., Hutton, I., Henmure, A. C. F., and Murdock, W. R. Hemodynamic and metabolic effects of hyperbaric oxygen in myocardial infarction. Lancet, October 15, 1966.

Chapman, C. B., Wright, I. S., and Hilden, T. Symposium on anticoagulants and coronary artery disease. Circulation, 30:444, 1961.

Datey, K. K., Hansoti, R. C., and Pandya, V. N. Value of fibrinolysin in management of myocardial infarction. J.A.M.A., 182:1078, 1962.

Deykin, D. Current concepts: the use of Heparin. New Eng. J. Med., 80:937, 1969.

Fletcher, G. F., Hurst, J. W., and Schlant, R. C. "Polarizing" solutions in patients with acute myocardial infarction. Amer. Heart J., 75:319, 1968.

Gifford, R. H., and Feinstein, A. R. Critique of studies of anticoagulant therapy for myocardial infarction. New Eng. J. Med., 280:351, 1969.

Hood, W. B., Yenikomshian, S., Norman, J. C., and Levine, H. D. Treatment of refractory ventricular tachysystole with hyperbaric oxygenation. Amer. J. Cardiol., 22:738, 1968.

Karell, P. De la cure de lait. Arch. Gen. Med., 118:513, 1866.

Langsjaen, P. H., Sanchez, S. A., Lynch, D. J., and Inman, T. W. The treatment of myocardial infarction with low molecular weight dextran. Amer. Heart J., 76:28, 1968.

Lown, B., and Sidel, V. W. Duration of hospital stay following acute myocardial infarction. Amer. J. Cardiol., 23:1, 1969.

Report by the M. R. C. Working Party. Potassium, glucose, and insulin treatment for acute myocardial infarction. Lancet, 2:1355, 1968.

Whalen, R. E., and Saltzman, H. A. Hyperbaric oxygenation in the treatment of acute myocardial infarction. Prog. Cardiovas. Dis., 10:575, 1968.

4

Oxygen Therapy in Acute Myocardial Infarction

The identification of the role of hypoxemia and alkalosis in the production of arrhythmia has led to one of the most significant advances in the treatment of myocardial infarction. Oxygen is a critical therapeutic agent in the treatment of acute myocardial infarction and yet it has been prescribed for decades with little scientific data to support or refute its use. Oxygen was prescribed empirically for cyanosis. Early studies showed that patients with an uncomplicated myocardial infarction had normal oxygen saturation, while those with pulmonary edema and shock were moderately desaturated. Not until arterial oxygen tension and pH were measured did the true significance of hypoxemia and alkalosis in "uncomplicated" myocardial infarction become manifest. The frequent association of hypoxemia and alkalosis has been clearly shown to initiate and propagate refractory ventricular and supraventricular arrhythmias in myocardial infarction.

Oxygen therapy has not always been stressed and has, in fact, been discouraged by some. While oxygen raises blood pressure and peripheral resistance, it may decrease cardiac output slightly. This has discouraged some from the use of oxygen in myocardial infarction. The critical role of alkalosis was not demonstrated in these early studies. We have studied the association of hypoxemia and alkalosis in a series of 45 patients admitted to the Coronary Care Unit for myocardial infarction (Table I). None of the patients had congestive heart failure or shock. Arterial gas analysis showed that the Po_2 averaged 58 mm Hg in 35 patients with proven transmural myocardial infarction, whereas those without infarction had Po_2 above 75 mm Hg. Respiratory alkalosis was observed in 11 of the 35 patients with myocardial infarction; two had mild metabolic acidosis.

TABLE 1. *Range and Average Values*

		pH	Po_2	O_2SAT	Pco_2	HCO_3
10 pts.	High	7.46	98.2	97.4	45.0	28.9
No AMI	Low	7.40	75.0	94.0	30.2	20.8
	Mean	7.425	85.68	95.73	38.64	24.82
	S.D.	.019	8.28	1.08	4.86	3.02
35 pts.	High	7.56	74.0	95.0	53.0	34.0
With AMI	Low	7.24	37.0	70.2	28.4	19.0
	Mean	7.43	58.44	88.29	36.62	24.70
	S.D.	.065	11.65	7.29	4.12	3.89

Gas Exchange Studies

Ventilation studies of 16 patients with transmural myocardial infarction were carried out. None of the patients were in overt congestive heart failure or shock. All were studied within 3 days of their admission to the Coronary Care Unit. All showed definite abnormalities. Pulmonary minute ventilation was increased in all cases. There was a significant gradient between the alveolar oxygen tension and arterial oxygen tension. The gradient of oxygen from alveolus to artery correlated positively with the elevation of the serum creatine phosphokinase (CPK). As the CPK rose, the gradient increased (Fig. 1). This probably represents a manifestation of left

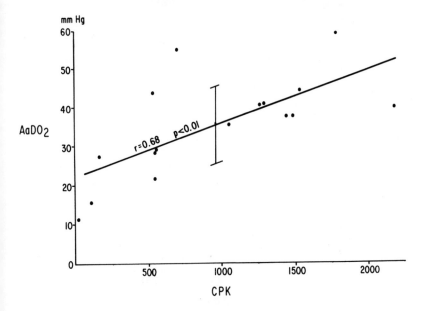

Creatine Phosphokinase & Hypoxemia in Myocardial Infarction

Fig. 1. The relationship between creatine phosphokinase (CPK) and arterial oxygen difference across the pulmonary bed (Aa DO_2). As the CPK rises indicating severity of infarcted myocardium, the Aa DO_2 increases indicating progressive hypoxemia. This means that the more severe the myocardial infarct, the greater is the hypoxemia.

ventricular dysfunction and markedly reduced cardiac output. Minute volume increases in an attempt to maintain normal oxygen tension. Arterial P_{CO_2} similarly correlated well with the rise in serum CPK (Fig. 2). As minute volume increased to maintain normal oxygen tension, the P_{CO_2} fell and was reflected by respiratory alkalosis.

The insult to the heart muscle from acute myocardial infarction results in diminished cardiac output. This inadequate cardiac output is manifested by hypoxemia (low P_{O_2}). It is partially compensated for by hyperventilation (low P_{CO_2}), with the resultant shift of the arterial pH toward alkalosis. These abnormalities are probably due to veno-arterial shunting of blood. The amount of blood through the shunt was calculated to be 9 percent of cardiac output. A noteworthy observation was that four maximal inflations reduced shunting from 9 to 6 percent of cardiac output. Our data place the cause of hypoxia

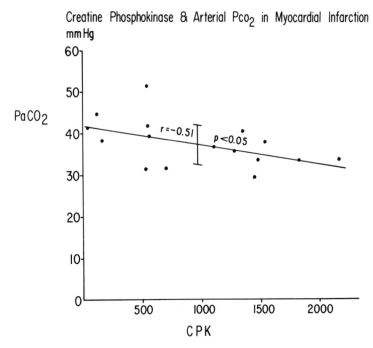

Fig. 2.   The relationship between CPK and arterial carbon dioxide tension (Pa CO_2). As the CPK rises the carbon dioxide tension decreases indicating alveolar hyperventilation. The hyperventilation is caused by hypoxemia and ultimately produces alkalosis.

on the basis of decreased cardiac output and pulmonary congestion. The compensation for hypoxemia is generally hyperventilation. Pulmonary engorgement from decreased cardiac output defeats this purpose and results in shunting of blood.

Hypoxemia may be further aggravated by the following: The oxyhemoglobin dissociation curve shifts to the left with alkalosis (Fig. 3). The normal curve shows a critically narrow band in the oxygen tension, where a modest reduction in Po_2 is associated with marked reduction in oxygen saturation. When alkalosis is present, the Po_2 may fall to very low levels with continued saturation of blood. Low oxygen tension intensifies tissue hypoxia by interfering with oxygen release in the capillary bed.

The failure to consider hypoxemia as a common problem in myocardial infarction stems from the clinician's failure to detect

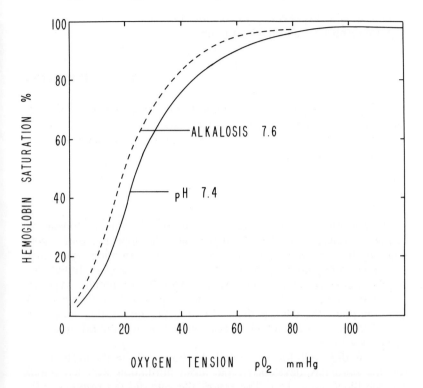

Fig. 3. Standard oxyhemoglobin dissociation curve. At low levels of oxygen tension the alkalotic patient may show relatively high oxygen saturation. The sigmoid curve is associated with wide changes in oxygen saturation in a narrow range of oxygen tension.

cyanosis. Reference to the oxyhemoglobin dissociation curve and to the oxygen saturation in the 35 patients with myocardial infarct shows that with alkalosis severe reductions in Po_2 may and does take place without unsaturation. Thus, cyanosis does not readily appear. Hypoxemia has been consistently observed in myocardial infarction by several investigators. If one waits until cyanosis appears, the hypoxemia is too far advanced.

The significance of alkalosis and arrhythmias can be seen. Based on five representative cases, it has been demonstrated that serious arrhythmias can be controlled by the correction of alkalosis alone without the need for anti-arrhythmic drugs. It has been further demonstrated that electrical and drug therapy fails in the presence of alkalosis and hypoxemia. Correction of these derangements may require respirators and tracheal intubation.

Case Reports

The following case reports indicate the value of proper oxygenation and ventilation in patients with arrhythmia. Some of these patients do not have acute myocardial infarction, but they illustrate the various points very well.

CASE 1*

A 77-year-old woman was transferred to St. Vincent's Hospital from a nursing home because of chest pain and the appearance of a pericardial friction rub. Diabetes mellitus, hypertension, pernicious anemia and hypothyroidism had been treated in the past. Initial electrocardiograms revealed sinus rhythm with left ventricular hypertrophy and ischemic ST-T waves over the left precordium. Enzyme studies confirmed the clinical diagnosis of acute myocardial infarction, although electrocardiographic evidence of a transmural infarction never developed.

She did well for the initial 48 hours of hospitalization, but on the third day developed rapid atrial fibrillation with left bundle branch block (Fig. 4A). The ventricular rate did not respond to 0.4 mg of ouabain, administered over 4 hours, so electrical conversion was attempted. A short period of asystole following the first countershock was followed by rapid atrial flutter with left bundle branch block (Fig. 4B). Quinidine sulfate, 400 mg I.M. was administered and repeated attempts at electrical conversion were made. Although sinus rhythm was generally restored, the patient quickly lapsed into rapid supraventricular tachycardia (Fig. 4C). Figure 4D shows the typical

* Conventional abbreviations are used, but the subscript for arterial location (lower case "a") has been omitted since all reference is to arterial sampling. Arterial blood was collected from patients in the CCU and in an Intensive Care Unit, and immediately delivered to the laboratory for analysis. Oxygen tension (Po_2) was determined by a microtip platinum electrode, and carbon dioxide tension (Pco_2) by a Severinghaus electrode. Methods of analysis, calibration and tonometry have been previously published. The samples were either analyzed immediately upon delivery to the laboratory or stored in a refrigerator. The maximum elapsed time between arterial sampling and analysis was one hour. (Cases 1-5 adapted from Ayres and Grace. Amer. J. Med., 46:495, 1969).

Atrial Fibrillation with LBBB

Atrial Flutter with LBBB

Intermittent Atrial Flutter

Onset of Atrial Flutter and
development of LBBB

Sustained Sinus Rhythm

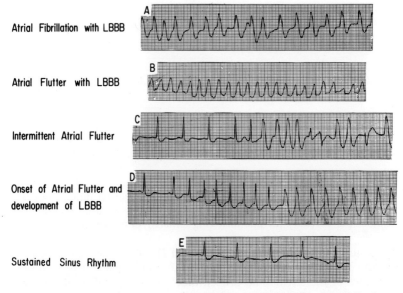

Fig. 4.   Representative tracings from Case 1 (see text). A and B show atrial fibrillation and atrial flutter with left bundle branch block (LBBB). C demonstrates repetitive nature of supraventricular arrhythmia, and D shows characteristic sequence of normal sinus rhythm replaced by atrial flutter with LBBB developing after seven normally conducted beats. Sustained sinus rhythm (E) was possible only after intubation and ventilation.

onset of atrial flutter following a period of sinus rhythm and the rate-related development of left bundle branch block. Propranolol, 3 mg I.V., and oral intubation finally produced a stable sinus bradycardia (Fig. 4E). Arterial blood gases were not obtained prior to intubation and ventilation with a pressure-cycled IPPB unit.

She remained in sinus rhythm on controlled ventilation and propranolol, 40 mg daily, until she pulled out her endotracheal tube. Her heart rate immediately slowed, changed to a junctional rhythm (Fig. 5), and then to rapid atrial flutter with left bundle branch block. She was immediately reintubated and returned spontaneously to sinus rhythm.

On the sixth day, she again developed rapid atrial fibrillation. Bedside ventilometer readings indicated a minute volume of 8.0 liter/min. and arterial studies were P_{O_2}, 77 mm Hg; P_{CO_2}, 22 mm Hg; pH, 7.51 units. Figure 6 demonstrates that she converted spontaneously to sinus rhythm as soon as the respiratory volume was decreased to 4.5

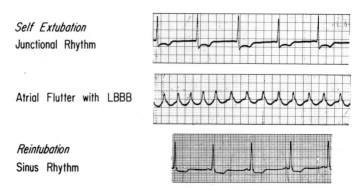

Self Extubation
Junctional Rhythm

Atrial Flutter with LBBB

Reintubation
Sinus Rhythm

Fig. 5. Junctional rhythm developed in Case 1 immediately after self-extubation and was followed in several minutes by atrial flutter with left bundle branch block. Sustained sinus rhythm was restored by reintubation without the necessity for administering antiarrhythmic agents.

liter/min. and the P_{CO_2} raised to 50 mm Hg. A further adjustment in minute volume lowered the P_{CO_2} to 33 mm Hg and led to disappearance of the left bundle branch block. Rapid atrial fibrillation recurred on the 13th day. Arterial studies revealed that she was well

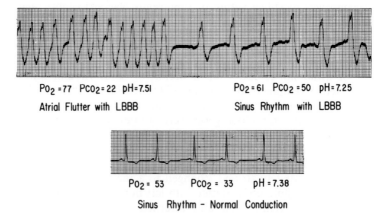

$P_{O_2} = 77$ $P_{CO_2} = 22$ pH = 7.51 $P_{O_2} = 61$ $P_{CO_2} = 50$ pH = 7.25

Atrial Flutter with LBBB   Sinus Rhythm with LBBB

$P_{O_2} = 53$ $P_{CO_2} = 33$ pH = 7.38

Sinus Rhythm - Normal Conduction

Fig. 6. Inadvertent hyperventilation produced respiratory alkalosis with atrial flutter and left bundle branch block. Bicarbonate concentration was 17.1 mEq per L at this time. Decreasing respiratory volume immediately led to sinus rhythm, but blood gas analysis revealed marked acidosis because of hypoventilation. A further adjustment in ventilation restored normal conduction as the pH was raised to 7.38. Hydrogen ion concentration is relatively high at all levels of P_{CO_2} because of the decrease in buffer base.

oxygenated (Po_2, 236 mm Hg), but that her Pco_2 was 17 mm Hg and her pH 7.63 units. Serum potassium was 3.1 mEq/liter. Five unsuccessful attempts at cardiac conversion had been made while the laboratory studies were being obtained. When the presence of severe respiratory alkalosis was appreciated, the respiratory volume was decreased and the patient spontaneously converted to sinus rhythm (Fig. 7). She remained in sinus rhythm and was gradually ambulated. On the 17th day, her Pco_2 was 33 mm Hg, pH, 7.45 units and Po_2, 55 mm Hg, breathing room air. Breathing 100 percent oxygen through a non-rebreathing system raised arterial Po_2 to 423 mm Hg and she was maintained on 40 percent oxygen administered by Puritan-heated nebulizer to her tracheostomy. Serum potassium was 4.3 mEq/liter.

On the 25th day, she was transferred from the Intensive Care Unit because of continued improvement. Several hours following transfer, she was found pulseless in bed, the tracheostomy tube having been pulled out and her airway occluded by secretions. Despite vigorous attempts at resuscitation, generalized brain damage was present and she died 24 hours later.

CASE 2

A 79-year-old man was admitted to St. Vincent's Hospital on September 27, 1967, with a presumed diagnosis of acute myocardial infarction and bilateral bronchopneumonia. On the 12th day, he was

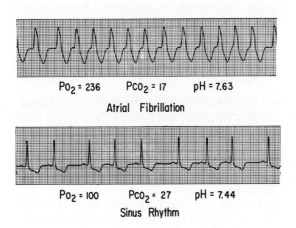

$Po_2 = 236$ $Pco_2 = 17$ pH = 7.63
Atrial Fibrillation

$Po_2 = 100$ $Pco_2 = 27$ pH = 7.44
Sinus Rhythm

Fig. 7. Hyperventilation in Case 1 again produced severe respiratory alkalosis which caused paroxysmal atrial fibrillation even though Po_2 was high. The patient converted to sinus rhythm as soon as respiratory volume was decreased.

noted to be in atrial flutter and was treated with sodium diphenyl-hydantoin (Dilantin), and two unsuccessful attempts at electrical conversion. He was found to be hypoxemic (Po_2, 50 mm Hg) and converted spontaneously to sinus rhythm following the elevation of Po_2 to 93 mm Hg with oxygen therapy. On the 15th day, atrial flutter recurred and was treated with both quinidine sulfate and countershock. In spite of intubation and four attempts at electrical conversion, atrial flutter persisted. Hypoxemia and alkalemia were both present (Po_2, 29 mm Hg; Pco_2, 23 mm Hg; and pH, 7.55 units). He was placed on a mechanical ventilator, sedated and returned to sinus rhythm. Following spontaneous conversion, blood gas studies revealed that Pco_2 had risen to 31 mm Hg and Po_2 to 60 mm Hg as a result of controlled mechanical ventilation.

On the 20th day, the patient was allowed to breathe spontaneously, but developed atrial flutter which was converted, following return to respirator therapy. Two subsequent episodes of atrial flutter responded to airway suctioning and assisted ventilation with the respirator. On the 27th day, while on the respirator, the patient became pulseless and was found to be in ventricular fibrillation. Attempts at resuscitation were unsuccessful until the tidal volume was decreased. Following decrease of tidal volume, a single precordial shock converted the patient to sinus rhythm. The patient had been ventilated at a rate of 17 liters per minute and was markedly alkalemic (Pco_2, 21 mm Hg; Po_2, 191 mm Hg and pH, 7.74 units); only a decrease in ventilation permitted restoration to sinus rhythm. His ventilation was carefully adjusted throughout his subsequent hospital course. He was gradually weaned from the respirator and remained in sinus rhythm.

CASE 3

A 51-year-old woman, brought to the Emergency Room with acute inferior wall infarction, was comatose at the time of hospital admission on April 21, 1967. The coma was presumed to be due to a period of asystole, due to Adams-Stokes attacks associated with the inferior infarction. Because of inability to breathe, the patient was placed on a pressure-cycled respirator and maintained on this unit for respiration thereafter.

From 2:45 P.M. on April 23, until 9:30 A.M. on April 24, 1967, the patient was electrically defibrillated on twenty-four separate occasions (Fig. 8A). At approximately this time, the blood gas levels were determined. They revealed a pH of 7.73 units and a Pco_2 of 13.3 mm Hg. Minute ventilation was 16 liters per minute. On the basis of these findings, the ventilation of the patient was changed to 6

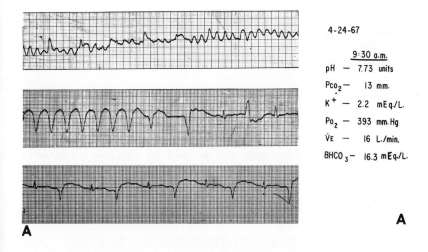

4-24-67

9:30 a.m.

pH — 7.73 units

Pco$_2$ — 13 mm.

K$^+$ — 2.2 mEq./L.

Po$_2$ — 393 mm.Hg

V̇E — 16 L./min.

BHCO$_3$ — 16.3 mEq./L.

A

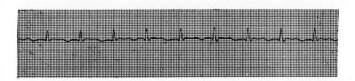

B

4-24-67

	10:30 a.m.		4 p.m.
pH —	7.54	units	7.47
Pco$_2$ —	29	mm.	33
K$^+$ —	2.7	mEq./L.	3.4
Po$_2$ —	143	mm.Hg	186
V̇E —	6	L./min.	5
BHCO$_3$ —	25.1	mEq./L.	23.5

Fig. 8. A variety of ventricular arrhythmias including ventricular fibrillation in response to a severe respiratory alkalosis produced by mechanical hyperventilation with a pressure cycled respirator (A). Marked hypokalemia and hypocapnia is shown in inset. Within minutes after readjusting the ventilator, Pco$_2$ and potassium rose, and there was a spontaneous conversion to sinus rhythm (B).

liters per minute. One hour later, at 10:30 A.M., the pH was 7.54 units and the patient was no longer having episodes of ventricular fibrillation (Fig. 8B). Thereafter there were no additional episodes of ventricular fibrillation; meticulous attention was paid to the ventila-ation of the patient and to control the serum pH.

The patient died suddenly on the sixth hospital day. Autopsy confirmed the diagnosis of inferior wall infarction.

CASE 4

A 60-year-old man was admitted to St. Vincent's Hospital for treatment of acute inferior infarction. From the time of admission to the hospital, the clinical course was marked by repeated episodes of supraventricular tachycardia and paroxysmal atrial fibrillation, as illustrated (Figs. 9A, 9B). The patient was treated with oxygen (nasal), digitalis and electrical cardioversion (four times) without

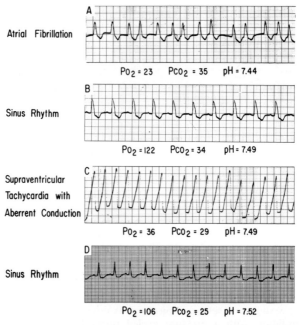

Fig. 9. Hypoxemia with a relatively normal pH led to repeated episodes of atrial fibrillation in Case 4 (A). Po_2 could not be adequately increased until the patient's beard was shaved and a tight mask fit achieved (B). Supraventricular tachycardia with aberrant conduction in Case 5 was due to severe hypoxemia and moderately severe respiratory alkalosis (C). Following intermittent positive pressure breathing therapy, sinus rhythm was restored, as Po_2 was raised to normal even though respiratory alkalosis persisted (D).

effect. The blood gases revealed a Po_2 of 56 mm Hg on the day of admission; arterial pH, 7.50 units. The patient was placed on a positive pressure respirator via face mask, but the Po_2 remained at 60 mm Hg, and the arrhythmia continued. This situation persisted throughout the first and second hospital days, when the patient noted that the mask he was using to breathe through did not fit very tightly. The patient had a heavy beard and he suggested that it was possible that the beard interfered with the fit of the mask. The beard was shaved, the patient was fitted with a tight mask and the Po_2 became 122 mm Hg. Within a few hours regular sinus rhythm appeared. He remained in sinus rhythm and intermittent positive pressure breathing was discontinued. On the sixth hospital day he developed rapid atrial fibrillation and was observed to have a severe respiratory alkalosis (Pco_2, 16 mm Hg; Po_2, 67 mm Hg; pH, 7.63 units). An endotracheal tube was passed and he was placed on a pressure-cycled respirator. After four hours, he returned to sinus rhythm. Blood gases were: pH, 7.55 units; Po_2, 140 mm Hg; Pco_2, 23 mm Hg.

CASE 5

A 64-year-old man was admitted to St. Vincent's Hospital for treatment of congestive heart failure and bronchopneumonia. The patient was in acute respiratory distress. Examination of the heart revealed S3 and S4 gallop rhythm, and moist rales were heard throughout the lungs.

At 10:00 A.M. on the day after admission, the patient began to have rapid supraventricular paroxysmal tachycardia with aberrant conduction (Fig. 9C). Intravenous lidocaine failed to control the arrhythmia. Intramuscular quinidine, two doses of 200 mg given one hour apart, and intravenous digoxin, 0.5 mg, failed to control the arrhythmia, which did respond transiently to carotid massage. From approximately noon that same day, almost constant attention to carotid massage resulted in only inadequate and infrequent control of the supraventricular paroxysmal tachycardia. The arterial oxygen tension at this time was 36 mm Hg, and the patient was given positive pressure oxygen by intermittent positive pressure breathing with a tightly fitting face mask. Approximately 3 minutes after a satisfactory adjustment of the face mask, and approximately at the same time that the arrhythmia was controlled, the Po_2 was 102 mm Hg (Fig. 9D).

COMMENT

This series of patients demonstrates that hypoxemia and alkalemia may produce serious atrial and ventricular arrhythmias and that only correction of the underlying metabolic abnormality can restore cardiac rhythm to normal. This combination, together with hypokalemia, appears to be the most common metabolic precursor of cardiac arrhythmias in the critically ill patient.

The frequency of alkalemia and hypoxemia in critically ill patients, their ubiquitous presence even in patients who appear clinically well, and their development from ventilation inappropriate to metabolic need have led us to the descriptive phrase "inappropriate pulmonary ventilation in the critically ill," simply for emphasis and teaching. The description implies that either hypo- or hyperventilation may seriously interfere with physiologic processes and attempts to remind the clinician to treat the resultant syndrome by appropriate means, rather than to continue the use of inappropriate drugs.

Hypoxemia is not the sole cause of alkalosis in acute myocardial infarction. After the correction of hypoxia, hyperventilation may persist in a number of patients. Other factors such as pain, anxiety, metabolic acidosis, and pulmonary congestion with stimulation of Hering-Breuer reflexes may cause hyperventilation. Sometimes the hyperventilation is so pronounced as to require the institution of controlled ventilation.

Methods of Oxygen Administration

Oxygen may be delivered to the patient by catheter, face mask, or through machines which can assist or control respiration. Each method of oxygen administration possesses special therapeutic advantages which will be discussed. The method of oxygen delivery should be tailored to the patient, but a broad outline of therapy may be drawn which embraces the majority. The following is our approach to the patient with acute myocardial infarction.

OXYGEN FOR THE ASYMPTOMATIC PATIENT

All patients receive oxygen by nasal cannula or face mask at a rate of 6-8 liters/minute. A double nasal cannula is preferred because it is well tolerated by most patients (Fig. 10). A face mask tends to interfere with simple taks, such as sipping water and eating. Most patients are intolerant of face masks and remove them (Fig. 11). In the absence of complications, oxygen is prescribed for the first 3 or 4

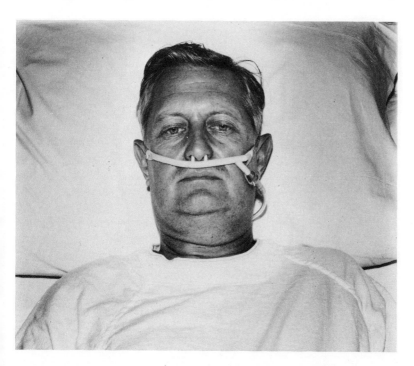

Fig. 10. A method of oxygen delivery which is acceptable to most patients. The nasal canulae extend one cm into the nose and cause very little discomfort.

days and then discontinued. In the presence of arrhythmias, shock, or congestive heart failure, oxygen is continued for 4 days after the complication is controlled, and arterial gas analysis is continuously monitored. Oxygen tents are no longer used in coronary care units, as they offer no more than local air conditioning and may be a hazard if electrical therapy for an arrhythmia is prescribed. Whenever increased oxygenation is required, assisted ventilation must be considered.

OXYGEN FOR ARRHYTHMIAS

Arrhythmias are treated first by administering oxygen. If an arrhythmia does not promptly disappear by giving oxygen by a nasal cannula or face mask, arterial blood is drawn to determine pH, Po_2, Pco_2 and HCO_3. Concurrently, oxygen is prescribed by inter-

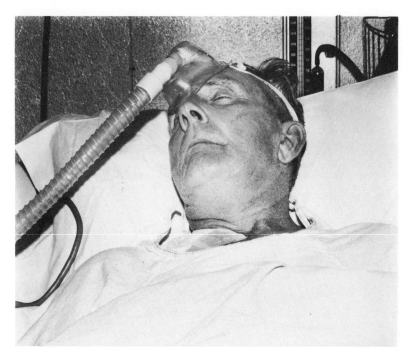

Fig. 11. The typical fate of oxygen masks. They provide 40 percent oxygen when properly fitted. However, masks are poorly tolerated by most patients and interfere with eating and drinking.

mittent positive pressure via face mask or oral piece. Generally, this is prescribed for 20 minutes and interrupted for 10 minutes. This is continued until the specific ventilatory abnormality based on the analysis of the arterial gas values is revealed. Ventilatory minute volume must be determined on every patient who requires assisted or controlled ventilation. Minute volume may be simply and accurately measured at the bedside with a ventilometer (Fig. 12). Estimating minute volume by observing the frequency and depth of respiration is erroneous and may lead to serious therapeutic errors.

　　Some arrhythmias respond to an elevation of the partial pressure of oxygen; most are due to respiratory alkalosis. Respiratory alkalosis is caused invariably by hyperventilation and it is this increase in minute volume which must be controlled in order to adjust pH toward normal. Hyperventilation may be reduced in several ways. Morphine sulfate in small doses, 6 to 8 mg subcutaneously, may be

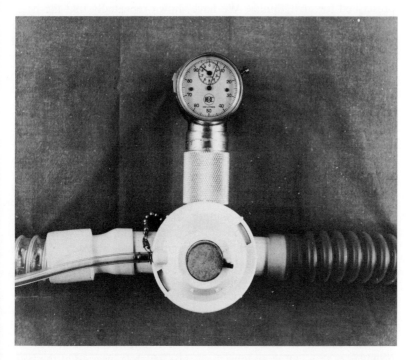

Fig. 12. A respirometer attached to the exhaust vent of a respirator. The meter is activated like a stop watch. Tidal volume and minute volume are measured in liters. Controlled ventilation must never be instituted without access to this simple device. No CCU should be without one.

prescribed while using an assisted positive pressure apparatus. Another technique consists in increasing the retard flow rate of a pressure-cycled respirator, thereby prolonging expiration. A third method is to increase inspiratory pressure so that the patient takes more time to trigger the apparatus and thereby prolong respiration. After manipulations are made to reduce the frequency of respiration, minute volume must be recorded at frequent intervals to assess the efficacy of therapy. Unless minute volume is reduced toward normal, alkalosis and arrhythmias cannot be controlled. Usually, it is not necessary to raise Po_2 to above 150 mm Hg. Prolonged ventilation with high concentration of oxygen may be hazardous. Oxygen, like other drugs, should be prescribed in sufficient quantities and not in excess.

Once the pH and hypoxemia are corrected, drug therapy may be prescribed for arrhythmias. We have shown repeatedly that the heart in a hypoxic and alkalotic milieu is less responsive to cardiotonic and anti-arrhythmic drugs. Cardioversion should never be attempted until all abnormalities of arterial gases are corrected. Defibrillation is often unsuccessful until acidosis and hypoxemia are corrected.

In summary, arrhythmias are treated by first correcting pH and hypoxemia. While anti-arrhythmic drugs are prescribed concomitantly, their efficacy is enhanced by correcting abnormalities in the cellular substrate.

CONTROLLED VENTILATION FOR SERIOUS COMPLICATIONS OF ACUTE MYOCARDIAL INFARCTION

An occasional patient cannot be oxygenated by the above method and control of complications (arrhythmia, shock, CHF) are seemingly impossible, even with extensive drug therapy. Such a patient must have his ventilation controlled with a respirator. The proper use of controlled ventilation is not a simple task and should never be contemplated without adequate facilities for constant monitoring of the arterial gases and for measuring minute volume. When controlled ventilation is used properly, the results may be dramatic.

In order to institute controlled ventilation, the patient must be provided with a cuffed endotracheal tube which is inserted at the bedside. The cuff is inflated with 5 cc of air. The endotracheal tube is connected to the respirator and a minute volume is prescribed which approaches normal, approximately 7 liters per minute. A true minute volume must be recorded with a ventilometer. Respirators are notoriously inaccurate in prescribing tidal volume. Errors of 5 percent in tidal volume are compounded in a minute and become staggering after several hours. This may lead to very serious alterations in acid-base balance. The only solution to this problem is to check the minute volume frequently with a ventilometer. After 15 minutes of controlled ventilation, a repeat analysis of arterial gas is made and compared with the baseline. Alterations may now be made in the minute volume, oxygen tension or bicarbonate stores. Once the appropriate minute volume is determined, arterial gas analysis should be determined twice per day.

Patients who do not immediately tolerate the endotracheal tube, or who continue to hyperventilate, must have their respiratory center controlled. Demerol, 10 mg intramuscular every hour, or alternating with Phenergan, 25 mg I.M., every hour, is usually sufficient to depress the respiratory center. Doses of Demerol as high as 50 mg per hour may have to be prescribed, but this is unusual. Controlled ventilation is continued until the related problem is solved. Arrhythmia is the common companion of respiratory alkalosis and usually responds to the control of alkalosis alone. Pulmonary edema, congestive heart failure, and shock are also accompanied by respiratory alkalosis, but in these cases correction of alkalosis alone, while beneficial, does not correct the underlying condition. Controlled ventilation adds to the management of pulmonary edema and congestive heart failure by diminishing the work of breathing, reducing venous return to the heart, and increasing intra-alveolar pressure.

Most patients tolerate an endotracheal tube very well. The tube is left in place for as long as 96 hours with no deleterious effect. The endotracheal tube has been left in place for longer periods, but this is not generally recommended. If a complication has not been controlled within 96 hours, a tracheostomy must be performed. We never perform tracheostomies as a primary approach for controlled ventilation. There has been some interest in nasotracheal tubes. These are uncomfortable, difficult to introduce and, in our experience, offer no more than endotracheal tubes.

HAZARDS OF CONTROLLED VENTILATION

The rapid control of alkalosis leads to prompt shifts in serum potassium concentration. Alkalosis leads to an efflux of potassium ion from the cells into the extracellular compartment. Sudden correction of alkalosis leads to a depletion of extracellular potassium. In the presence of digitalis, this may be lethal.

Disconnection of the respirator from the endotracheal tube may occur and lead to asphyxia. Since the respiratory center is paralyzed to control ventilation, apnea and death will occur if the respirator is disconnected. The solution to this problem is to install an apnea alarm in the respirator. This is triggered by a sudden fall in inspiratory pressure (if the machine is disconnected from the endotracheal tube). An Ambu bag should always be available in emergency.

Separation of the cuff from the tracheostomy tube: fortunately, this accident no longer happens, since the abandonment of tracheostomies. Endotracheal tubes are incorporated with a cuff that cannot be detached.

False central venous pressures: A positive pressure respirator must be disconnected while recording central venous pressure.

Ulceration of the vocal cords: This is a rare complication when endotracheal tubes are prescribed for not longer than 96 hours. It seems prudent to deflate the cuff periodically in order to prevent tracheal ulceration. The nasopharynx should first be aspirated of secretions in order to prevent aspiration.

CONCLUDING REMARKS

Oxygen is critical to the patient with acute myocardial infarction and should be prescribed for all patients, no matter how well they may appear clinically. When patients experience complications such as arrhythmias, shock or congestive heart failure, an appropriate system of delivering oxygen should be prescribed. The basis for the amount prescribed is the assessment of respiratory minute volume, the analysis of arterial gases, and the determination of serum electrolytes.

References

Ayres, S. M., and Grace, W. J. Inappropriate ventilation and hypoxemia as causes of cardiac arrhythmias. Amer. J. Med., 46:495, 1969.

Hardy, W. E., Ayres, S. M., Keyloun, V. E., and Grace, W. J. Causes of hypoxemia and alkalemia in acute myocardial infarction. Clin. Research, 16: 370, 1968

Keyloun, V. E., Ayres, S. M., and Grace, W. J. Hypoxemia in acute myocardial infarct (abstract). Clin. Research, 15:450, 1967.

Lal, S., Savige, R. S., and Chabra, G. P. Oxygen administration after myocardial infarction. Lancet, 1:381, 1969.

MacKenzie, G. J., et al. Circulatory and respiratory studies in myocardial infarction and shock. Lancet, 2:825, 1964.

McNicol, M. W., et al. Pulmonary function in acute myocardial infarction. Brit. Med. J., 2:1270, 1965.

Neill, W. A. Myocardial hypoxia and anaerobic metabolism in coronary heart disease. Amer. J. Cardiol., 22:507, 1968.

Shillingford, J. P., and Thomas, M. Cardiovascular and pulmonary changes in patients with myocardial infarction treated in an intensive care and research unit. Amer. J. Cardiol., 20:484, 1967.

Thomas, M., Malmcrona, R., Fillmore, S., and Shillingford, J. Haemodynamic effects of morphine in patients with acute myocardial infarction. Brit. Heart J., 27:863, 1965.

Valentine, A., and Burgess, J. H. Arterial hypoxemia following acute myocardial infarction. Circulation, 50:641, 1969.

Valentine, P. A., et al. Blood gas changes after acute myocardial infarction. Lancet, 2:837, 1966.

Wildenthal, K., Fuller, D. S., and Shapiro, W. Paroxysmal atrial arrhythmias induced by hyperventilation. Amer. J. Cardiol., 21:436, 1968.

5

Arrhythmias in Acute Myocardial Infarction

Arrhythmia in acute myocardial infarction was thought to be the most frequent cause of death. Before the institution of the Coronary Care Unit system for the management of patients with acute myocardial infarction, it was generally stated that the causes of death in this condition were:

Arrhythmia	70%	
Shock	10%	
Heart Failure	10%	(pulmonary embolism, rupture
Other	10%	of ventricle, etc.)

Significantly, these arrhythmias in the main are treatable.

The arrhythmias detected at cardiac arrest in St. Vincent's Hospital prior to continuous monitoring were as follows:

Ventricular fibrillation	51
Asystole	32
Complete heart block	9
Sinus bradycardia	3
Chaotic rhythm	11
Not recorded	2

Although such data derived from experience in the period prior to continuous ECG monitoring are open to some objection, we feel this information is reliable and useful.

The Coronary Care Unit was originally conceived to facilitate resuscitation. However, it soon became apparent that continuous ECG monitoring and the diagnosis and treatment of arrhythmia, before cardiac arrest, was to be the prime effort of the Coronary Care Unit. Consideration of cumulative data from the Coronary Care Unit provides the following distribution of the causes of death.*

Ventricular fibrillation	12%
Ventricular standstill	20%
Shock	30%
Congestive heart failure	20%
Unknown, miscellaneous	18%

The apparent increase in shock and heart failure are simply reflections of the reduction in deaths due to arrhythmia. This reduction is due to the endless search of the ECG monitors for the "early signs of the life-threatening arrhythmia" and their prompt treatment.

The reduction in mortality from acute myocardial infarction has been due mainly to control of cardiac arrhythmia (See Chapter 1, Table 12). *"The name of the game is arrhythmia."*

The Danger to the Patient in Cardiac Arrhythmia

The patient with acute myocardial infarction has substantial damage to the cardiac muscle resulting in a lowering of the cardiac

---

* Based on 625 patients at St. Vincent's Hospital.

output. Additionally, the cardiac output is lowered by two other mechanisms: 1) alteration in the ventricular rate; and 2) alteration in cardiac rhythm. Although these are frequently found together, as in rapid atrial fibrillation, the abnormality of rate or the abnormality of the A-V conduction may be separable.

Cardiac output and aortic pressure determine the coronary flow and myocardial perfusion. Hence, a vicious cycle may be established. Myocardial infarction results in a lowered cardiac output and lowered aortic pressure. These in turn further reduce perfusion of the coronary arteries and myocardium. This reduction in the oxygenation of the myocardium may result in an arrhythmia and further deterioration of function.

Cardiac Output and Heart Rate

The cardiac output in general is closely related to ventricular rate. The pumping mechanism of the heart functions most efficiently between well-defined limits. Heart rates between 60 and 110 beats per minute have been shown to be the most efficient in terms of cardiac output, oxygen consumption, and lactate metabolism of the myocardium. Within wide limits, then, the cardiac output is determined by the ventricular rate. Arrhythmias that are characterized by, or associated with, extremes of rate are dangerous. The cardiac output falls precipitously at slow ventricular rates (below 40 to 50) and it falls similarly at high rates (120 to 140 or higher).

Bradyarrhythmias or A-V dissociation with slow ventricular rates and tachyarrhythmias with rapid ventricular rates are examples of rate disturbances affecting the cardiac output. Although there is no definite laboratory evidence, there are strong feelings among clinicians that the patient with acute myocardial infarction tolerates arrhythmias far less well than does the random population.

Cardiac Output in A-V Dissociation, Atrial Fibrillation and Flutter

A decline of 25 percent in the cardiac output is noted in rhythm disturbances, such as A-V dissociation, atrial fibrillation or atrial flutter. This decline is attributable to the A-V dissociation alone. The

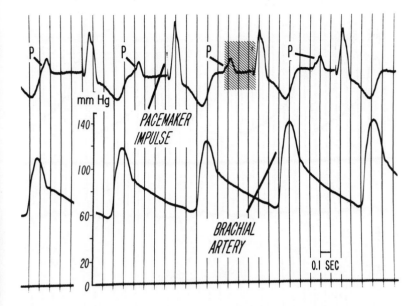

Fig. 1. The effect of atrial contraction on central blood pressure. When atrial contraction (shaded area) falls in its proper place in the cardiac cycle the arterial pressure is 20 mm Hg greater. The results were recorded from a patient with a fixed-rate pacemaker. Note that the P-R interval of the first and second beat is abnormal and thus contributes little to central blood pressure. (Adapted from Ayres and Giannelli. *Care of the Critically Ill*, 1967. Courtesy of Appleton-Century-Crofts.)

reduction is due to the loss of the atrial contraction (atrial "kick"), as in atrial fibrillation, or to improper timing of the atrial contraction in the cardiac cycle, as in A-V dissociation. This, although a rather modest loss of cardiac output, may be critical to some patients whose cardiac output has already been greatly reduced by other factors (Fig. 1).

Cardiac Output in Rapid Ventricular Rates

Pulsus alternans is often noted in rapid ventricular rates. When pulsus alternans is present, the stroke volume is low in those beats with the small pulse, or the beat with the lower ECG amplitude (Fig. 2). Almost any rhythm disturbance can be tolerated if the ventricular rate remains within reasonable limits (50 to 120). Some persons tend

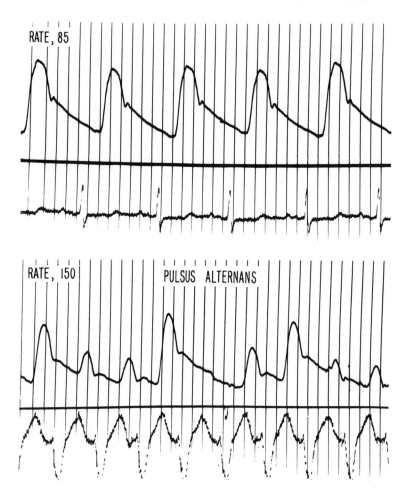

Fig. 2. Pulse pressure curves are recorded at normal rates. When heart rate accelerates in the presence of myocardial damage pulsus alternans is recorded, with subsequent lowering of the blood pressure and presumably of the cardiac output. Rapid rate was recorded while a pacemaker was being adjusted. (Adapted from Ayres and Giannelli. *Care of the Critically Ill,* 1967. Courtesy of Appleton-Century-Crofts.)

to have a falling cardiac output with ventricular rates of 110 beats per minute, whereas others may reach 150 before the cardiac output significantly falls. In any event, the cardiac output tends to fall as the rate increases to the higher ranges (120 to 140). This may be due in part to the short diastolic ventricular filling time, so that stroke output

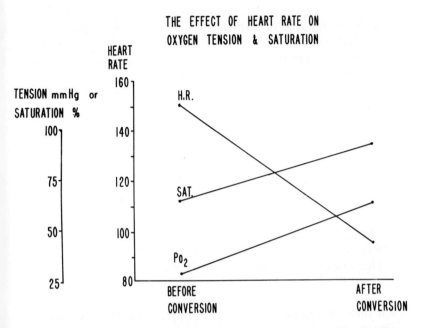

Fig. 3. The relationship of rapid heart rate on arterial gas analysis. When the heart is in atrial flutter with a ventricular rate of 150 beats per minute, both oxygen tension and saturation are abnormally low. Within minutes after electric conversion of the arrhythmia, oxygen tension and saturation return to normal. Oxygen was not administered during this study.

is greatly reduced. Tachycardia also increases O_2 consumption of the myocardium out of proportion to the cardiac output (Fig. 3 illustrates the inability of the patient to oxygenate himself during rapid ventricular rates).

These comments on the effects of arrhythmia on cardiac output are emphasized to bring home the concept that, in treating the arrhythmias, we are aiming to correct or prevent a falling cardiac output which results from their continuance.

The Life-Threatening Arrhythmias

Arrhythmias are present in 80 to 90 percent of patients with acute myocardial infarction. These high figures represent all deviations

from normal sinus rhythm, including those which appear only transiently. Not every type of arrhythmia is serious. Some appear briefly
and terminate spontaneously. Others represent a significant departure
from normal and are potentially serious. These are referred to as the
life-threatening arrhythmias, which are as follows:

1) Tachyarrhythmias:
   Ventricular— 1) ventricular premature beat
                2) ventricular tachycardia
                3) ventricular flutter and fibrillation
   Atrial   — 1) atrial premature beats
                2) atrial ectopic tachycardia
                3) atrial flutter
                4) atrial fibrillation
2) Bradyarrhythmias:
   Sinus Bradycardia (ventricular rate below 50)
   Heart Block 2° with slow ventricular rate
   Heart Block 3° with slow ventricular rate

When such arrhythmias are detected, appropriate therapy must be
instituted promptly.

Generally speaking, the tachyarrhythmias are associated with
anterior wall infarction, and the bradyarrhythmias and heart block
with inferior wall infarction.

If the patient can be carried past the first few critical days, the
arrhythmias generally disappear. In most instances, the conduction
system is not permanently damaged and the irritable ectopic foci
become either fully viable or heal by fibrosis. Autopsy studies of
patients who die of arrhythmias have confirmed the integrity of the
conduction system. The acute episode which causes the arrhythmia,
once corrected, results in normal conduction and rhythm.

The arrhythmias in myocardial infarction which are treatable
and correctable are those associated primarily with electrical instability of the heart. Recently, they have been referred to as *electrical failure*. They are to be distinguished from the arrhythmias which may
accompany congestive heart failure and shock. Correction of the
arrhythmias associated with the latter condition does not, as a rule,
increase survival. Arrhythmias in patients with congestive heart failure may be responsible for the heart failure itself and correction of
these may be life-saving. However, the occurrence of severe heart

failure or acute pulmonary edema indicates a very serious state, the control of which may depend upon many factors other than the control of the arrhythmia.

The Diagnosis of Arrhythmia

Proper therapy of an arrhythmia depends on proper diagnosis. Although some arrhythmias may be diagnosed by clinical means (atrial fibrillation), electrocardiographic diagnosis is essential for precise classification. In order to diagnose an arrhythmia, the following are necessary:

1) an *adequate* electrocardiograph;
2) a systematic interpretation;
3) a pair of calipers.

These will be discussed separately.

1. *An adequate electrocardiograph.* For this purpose, an adequate ECG is defined as one that clearly shows atrial activity (P waves, or flutter waves, or fibrillation waves). Commonly, a long Lead II and/or V_1 is obtained. All too often, however, such "rhythm" strips fail to display the atrial activity and additional steps are then necessary to prevent an endless discussion about tiny bumps and valleys in the graph:

Then—

a) All twelve leads are taken.

b) Leads showing atrial activity most clearly are recorded while one or the other carotid sinus (but not both simultaneously) is massaged. This may produce a degree of A-V block, revealing the basic atrial rhythm (Fig. 4).

c) A Lewis lead is recorded if P waves are not readily observed in the standard electrocardiogram. The Lewis lead is made by taking the right arm wire (negative) and attaching it to the second right interspace parasternally by the usual chest lead suction cup. The left arm lead (positive) is similarly attached to the chest wall at the fourth interspace to the right of the sternum. Lead I on the ECG machine should be used. The left arm lead can then be used to locate the P vector by moving it inch by inch, leftward and upward, toward the patient's left nipple. Other locations can be explored (Fig. 5).

d) An esophageal lead may be necessary. An especially constructed lead wire is introduced into the esophagus to the level of the

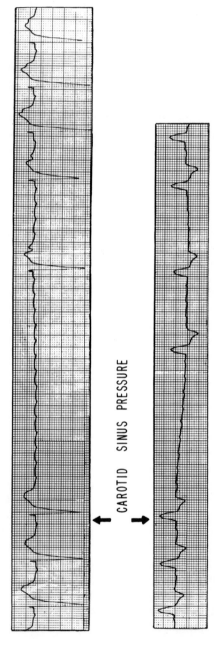

CAROTID SINUS PRESSURE

Fig. 4. The effect of carotid sinus pressure is demonstrated by a slowing of ventricular rate. The first three complexes in each rhythm strip appear to be preceded by a P wave. The apparent sinus rhythm is shown to be atrial flutter only after carotid sinus pressure is applied.

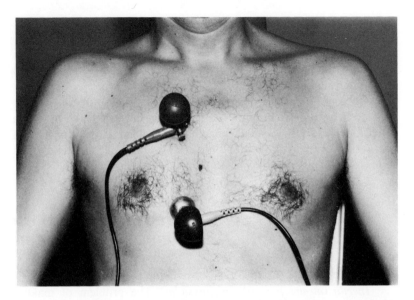

Fig. 5. A Lewis lead, employed to demonstrate P waves, is recorded by attaching the right arm lead wire at the second interspace to the right of the sternum and the left arm lead wire at the fourth interspace to the right of the sternum by means of suction cups. The ECG lead selector is placed at Lead I. The lower suction cup may be advanced toward the left nipple until a suitable P wave is recorded.

atrium. The other end is attached to the chest lead wire. P waves recorded by such techniques are frequently larger than the QRS. Hence, it may be important to have the standard leads recorded before and after, or simultaneously, with the esophageal lead in order to be able to identify the complexes.

2. *A system of interpretation.* The text, *Clinical Electrocardiography—The Arrhythmias,* by Pick and Katz, is used as a basis of reference. The systematic approach taught in this text is particularly important in interpreting the slow arrhythmias, various types of heart block, and the complex arrhythmias.

3. *A pair of calipers.* One cannot read an electrocardiogram without *using a pair of calipers* and systematically pacing out the various complexes. The use of pencil marks for the various complexes on the sides of a small piece of paper, the "prescription blank method," is simply not adequate. There are no short cuts to interpretation. Electrocardiographic strips (2 or 3 feet long at least) must be placed

on a flat surface with good lighting and evaluated with the calipers. First, find the P wave, then determine if the P waves are evenly spaced. Demonstrate with the caliper whether the QRS intervals are regular or not, and that the relationship between the P waves and QRS is constant or not.

Once the diagnosis of arrhythmia is established, treatment may proceed in an orderly fashion. Confident steps may be taken based on exact knowledge. It is more economical to spend a few moments in diagnosing an arrhythmia along carefully worked out principles than to make costly assumptions based on incomplete information.

What Interferes With Prompt Treatment of Arrhythmias?

Inertia on the part of the physician. The problem of making decisions is always difficult. A wrong decison on the part of the physician is unacceptable, even if the therapy undertaken does no harm. For example, inserting a transvenous pacemaker which is not used. Part of the gamesmanship of the modern-day house officer is to see how far he can go and still "get away with it." Patients cannot tolerate life-threatening arrhythmias, even if the doctor can. Action to control an arrhythmia must be started just as soon as it is diagnosed. No harm is done if medication is placed in an intravenous infusion and later discontinued. The only possible harm is the ridicule of one's associates. The problem of placing an intravenous pacemaker in a patient who is having convulsions, or who is in shock, is fraught with overwhelming difficulties compared to placing the catheter before a crisis arises. We wish to urge the "aggressive treatment of arrhythmia" and the prevention of life-threatening arrhythmia by early detection and treatment of all arrhythmias.

The availability of the physician. This ultimately may prove to be the crux to the success of coronary care units. Most coronary care units during the early stage of development showed little improvement in survival rates because therapy waited for the arrival of the physician. Only when nurses were taught to institute treatment in the absence of the physician did mortality rates fall. In the smaller hospital without a physician on hand, the backbone of the coronary care unit is the nurse. Unless she is trained to detect and treat arrhythmias, the survival rate will not be improved.

Training the team. Instituting resuscitative procedures, defibrillation or cardiac massage can be a harrowing experience to the uninitiated physician or nurse. A system of training to keep the medical team razor sharp must be developed within each coronary care unit, so that any member of the team can defibrillate a patient in the shortest possible time. One such system is to practice on anesthetized dogs on a weekly basis (see page 207). Football players scrimmage between games—why should the medical team not practice between challenges? Put another way—the troops must be kept in practice.

Plan of therapy. While every patient should be considered individually, certain arrhythmias demand immediate care. The appearance of ventricular premature beat should not produce a conference, but action. Complete heart block should not be the topic of debate, but calls for the immediate implantation of a temporary transvenous pacemaker. Theoretic discussions should be carried out before the life-threatening arrhythmias appear. Be prepared to act.

The Electrical Management of Arrhythmias (Technical Aspects)

While some arrhythmias are altered by oxygen and drug therapy, many life-threatening arrhythmias respond promptly to one of three electrical therapeutic modalities. They are:

1) electric cardioversion;
2) electric defibrillation;
3) electric pacemakers.

The technique of applying these forms of treatment will be explicitly described and referred to in the discussion of treatment of the specific arrhythmias.

ELECTRICAL CARDIOVERSION— DIRECT CURRENT COUNTERSHOCK— ESSENTIALS OF THE APPARATUS AND PROCEDURES

Electric cardioversion effects instant and total depolarization of the heart. Theoretically an ectopic or circus movement is halted by total depolarization permitting the more normal pacemakers to take over cardiac rhythm. Cardioversion is achieved by delivering a pre-scribed dose of direct current,* measured in watt-seconds, at a pre-cise time in the cardiac cycle (the downstroke of the R wave). Elec-tronic equipment has reduced this complex procedure to the selection of a few dials and pushing a button. Every machine presently avail-able is equipped with standard parts which vary little from unit to unit.

Selection of the Proper Lead in Cardioversion

A conventional electrocardiogram will quickly demonstrate the lead with the tallest R wave. Lead wires from the cardioverter are attached to the patient's extremities or chest wall in such a manner as to approximate the ECG lead with the tallest R wave. The R wave on the oscilloscopic screen of the cardioverter must be 2 cm tall so that the machine will not confuse the R wave with a tall T wave. When the T wave is as tall as the QRS complex, the lead selected should be abandoned and another chosen to reduce the possibility of error. The electronic devices do not distinguish between T waves and R waves. When an R wave at least 2 cm tall is not recorded, the amplifiers enlarge the QRS electrically by an "amplitude" dial on some machines or "V" gain on others.

Dose Selector

The amount of electricity which is used to convert heart rhythms is measured in watt-seconds.

$$Watt = volts \times amps$$
$$Watt\text{-}second = watt \times time$$

The dose ranges from one to 400 watt-seconds. Doses as little as one watt-second have been known to convert atrial flutter. Doses above 400 watt-seconds are never prescribed because of the production of severe burns to the chest wall. Similar to drug therapy the lowest effective dose of electricity is prescribed. For most cases of atrial fibrillation or atrial tachycardia, 150 to 250 watt-seconds usually suf-

---

* Alternating current defibrillators are no longer in general use.

fice. Atrial flutter responds generally to lower doses (50 watt-seconds for the first trial). If the patient has been taking digitalis, start with 25 watt-seconds. If the patient is thought to be digitalis-toxic, do *not* cardiovert.

THE ELECTRODES (PADDLES)

The electricity is delivered through two circular paddles. They are placed on the chest wall so that the electric current flows through the heart and not around it. The heart lies in the thoracic cage surrounded by the poorly conducting air-filled lungs. Electricity, like water, follows the path of least resistance. If the paddles are placed too close to each other, electricity will flow from one to the other through the skin and muscle of the chest wall and never reach the heart; if placed too far apart the electric current will be dissipated. The V_1 and V_6 positions have been shown to be effective. Rarely do the paddles need to be positioned so that one lies posteriorly at the base of the left scapula and the other placed anteriorly at the V_3 position. The paddles are applied to the chest wall with firm pressure (about 15 lb./sq. inch) after being thoroughly coated with electrode jelly. Too much jelly applied to the chest wall may cause an electric arc between the paddles and short-circuit the path of electricity away from the heart. Uneven pressure applied to the paddles may similarly produce an arc causing severe skin burns.

ANESTHESIA FOR ELECTRIC CARDIOVERSION

General anesthesia is unnecessary. During the infancy of cardioversion, patients were anesthetized with intravenous pentobarbital. There was little deleterious effect. Valium is presently the drug of choice. It affords total amnesia with little risk of hypotension in the dose of 5 mg administered intravenously and repeated in 2 minutes if necessary. When the patient fails to respond to his name or some simple command, he is ready to be cardioverted. Narcosis is not necessary when using Valium.

Cardioversion produces a momentary pain, which may awaken the patient and cause him to cry out, but rarely is there any recollection of the event. The patient usually falls asleep for from 1 to 2 hours afterward. Intubation is not necessary. Oxygen is administered during the height of narcosis by means of an Ambu bag but not during the act of cardioversion.

Generally, with the supraventricular tachycardias one likes to wait for 4 hours after the last meal before giving the anesthesia. However, some cardiac crises such as ventricular tachycardia or fibrillation or atrial tachycardia with falling blood pressure demand immediate cardioversion. Cardioversion has been carried out under such circumstances without anesthesia or narcosis. There has been surprisingly little complaint from patients under these circumstances. Cardioversion without anesthesia is reserved for those special clinical situations which demand it. Precious time should not be wasted waiting for narcosis or anesthesia.

PREMEDICATION FOR ELECTRIC CARDIOVERSION

For elective cardioversion, patients are kept fasting for 4 hours. Quinidine gluconate, 400 mg I.M., is prescribed at least 2 hours before cardioversion. This accomplishes two things: 1) quinidine itself aborts or converts about 40 percent of supraventricular tachyarrhythmias; 2) quinidine suppresses the ectopic focus after cardioversion and helps to maintain sinus rhythm. A maintenance dose of 200 mg, orally every 6 hours, is prescribed until the clinical situation justifies discontinuance. Accelerated ventricular rates (atrial flutter with 1:1 conduction) are rarely encountered with a premedicating dose of quinidine. If it occurs the patient is promptly cardioverted (Fig. 6).

PREPARATION OF PATIENT FOR ELECTRIC CARDIOVERSION

Before any attempt is made to convert an arrhythmia, two abnormalities must be corrected if they exist: 1) acidosis, and 2) hypoxemia. The heart in metabolic acidosis is resistant to the conversion of any arrhythmia. Adequate sodium bicarbonate should be administered to correct acidosis. Hypoxemia is less easily corrected in the face of an arrhythmia. Nevertheless, the patient should be ventilated and assisted using an Ambu bag prior to cardioversion. In elective cases patients whose ECG suggests digitalis excess or who have other manifestations of digitalis toxicity should not be electrically cardioverted until the digitalis has been discontinued for at least 48 hours.

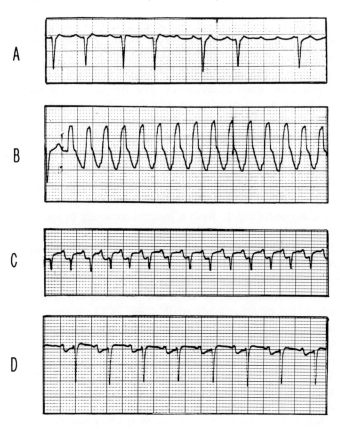

Fig. 6. Quinidine is prescribed for atrial flutter with varying A-V block (A). After one-half hour the patient developed a supraventricular tachycardia with bundle branch block (B) which was defined as atrial flutter with 1:1 A-V conduction (C). Paradoxic accelerated ventricular rates are immediately cardioverted (D) with D-C countershock. (All rhythm strips are lead V_1).

POSTCARDIOVERSION ARRHYTHMIA

Immediately after cardioversion many patients develop atrial arrhythmias, especially atrial premature contractions. Sometimes nodal rhythm will occur transiently. First degree A-V block is frequently seen. These arrhythmias do not last more than a few minutes and are not troublesome. Rarely, nodal rhythm persists for a few days, usually at a slow rate.

In some patients it is advisable to insert a transvenous pacemaker before attempting cardioversion, especially when serious disease is suspected in the A-V node, manifested by previous episodes of a high degree of block or previous episodes of junctional rhythm or episodes of slow sinus bradycardia. The typical clinical situation is represented by a patient with an inferior wall infarction who developed atrial flutter with a slow ventricular rate. Conversion may result in very slow ventricular rate. Caution should be exercised by having the pacemaker wire inserted beforehand. Similarly, the patient with a wandering atrial pacemaker who then develops atrial fibrillation should have an electric pacemaker catheter inserted before conversion is attempted. While slow nodal rhythms rarely develop after cardioversion it is comforting to have a pacemaker ready to speed the ventricular rate when indicated.

Step-by-step procedure: After being sure that the patient is well oxygenated and is not acidotic,

1. attach patient to standard electrocardiograph;
2. from the standard ECG select the lead with tallest R wave;
3. attach the monitor leads so that the ECG on the oscilloscope approximates the lead with the tallest R wave;
4. select prescribed dose (watt-seconds);
5. administer Valium 5 mg I.V. Repeat once if necessary;
6. assist respiration with Ambu bag and oxygen;
7. apply electrode paste to paddles;
8. apply paddles to chest wall at V_1 and V_5;
9. command all assistants not to touch the bed (say in a loud clear voice, "Everybody—off the bed!");
10. disconnect ECG wire from machine momentarily;
11. cardiovert. The code word is "Hit it!";
12. replace ECG wire in machine and record continuous rhythm strip;
13. record BP every 2 minutes until stable;
14. if the abnormal rhythm returns, cardiovert again using higher current. If normal rhythm persists for 2 to 3 minutes, it will persist in all probability;
15. turn the machine off. The DC cardioverter has a capacitor which builds a store of electricity within moments of discharge. That is to say the machine recharges immediately. The dose selector should be turned to zero and with the paddles widely separated the machine discharged. Failure to do so may result in an accidental electrocution or fire.

HAZARDS AND THERAPY

In the construction of a new coronary care unit electrical engineers should provide for a common ground wire separate from that of the rest of the hospital. This prevents "leakage" and electric catastrophes. In older construction, blocks of AC outlets are grounded separately. In one room the ground wires of separate electric outlets might be unequal. This creates a potential setting for a catastrophe: for example, a monitor and cardioverter on one outlet and an electrocardiograph machine on another outlet with unequal grounds permit 60 cps current to "leak" from one machine to another and cause ventricular fibrillation or serious burn to the patient. The best prevention is to accept nothing but the best wiring system available. If there is any question about the electric circuitry, all machines should be plugged into the same battery of AC outlets and grounded jointly to the earth or a cold water pipe. At the moment of cardioversion the patient cable to the electrocardiograph machine should be disconnected; otherwise the machine may be burned out by the high voltage from the cardioverter. This momentary disconnection will permit the recording of heart beat immediately after conversion. Failure to do so results in a delay of several minutes until the ECG machine recovers from the high voltage electrical input.

FAILURE TO CARDIOVERT

1. Increase dose in increments of 50 watt-seconds to maximum of 400 watt-seconds.
2. Correct acidosis or alkalosis if present.
3. Correct hypoxemia.
4. Re-evaluate the arrhythmia for accuracy of diagnosis.

INDICATIONS FOR CARDIOVERSION

In acute myocardial infarction the following arrhythmias should be promptly cardioverted:
1. Ventricular tachycardia, flutter and fibrillation.
2. Atrial flutter.
   The following arrhythmias should be cardioverted if associated with rapid ventricular rates or falling blood pressure:
1. Atrial fibrillation.

2. Atrial tachycardia.

These will be discussed separately and in detail in the section on arrhythmia.

CARDIOVERSION OF THE PATIENT TAKING DIGITALIS

See various arrhythmias (pp. 89, 108, and 141) as special caution is required.

Cardiac Pacemakers— Technical Aspects

There are two types of pacemaker wires available—unipolar and bipolar—and two methods of pacing the heart—at a fixed rate and "on demand." Unipolar wires are tiny and filamentous. They can be introduced easily into a vein through a large bore needle so that venous cutdown is unnecessary. The disadvantage of the unipolar wires is the placement of the second electrode. This is usually fixed to the chest wall and results in contraction of the pectoralis or underlying muscle whenever the heart is paced, which is a troublesome feature poorly tolerated by most patients. The bipolar electrode, with rare exceptions, is used exclusively. It consists of two platinum-tipped wires wrapped in a polyethylene sheath. When the wire is placed adjacent to the myocardium, electric current passes from one platinum tip to another through the heart muscle, thereby stimulating it and causing it to contract. Bipolar pacemaker wires are durable, safe and reusable (gas sterilization is recommended).

The two methods of pacing the heart are fixed rate and demand type. As the term implies, fixed rate pacing means that the battery-powered source of pacemaker energy is all or none. The machine is either on or off, both the rate and voltage being unvariable. Once the pacemaker is on it continues to "pace" regardless of cardiac rhythm. This type of pacing is eminently suitable for Adams-Stokes disease due to permanent complete heart block and slow ventricular rates. This was the first type to be developed and gained wide acceptability. However, many patients in heart block revert to sinus or some other supraventricular rhythm. The fixed rate pacemaker then competes with the inherent cardiac pacemakers and sometimes results in interference and even death due to pacemaker discharge during the vulnerable period of the T wave. We no longer use fixed rate pacemakers (Fig. 7).

Demand pacemakers are an engineering breakthrough and result in a more physiologic approach to the problem of heart block. The battery-powered source is programmed to discharge when it fails to "detect" a QRS complex within a specific period of time. Thus if the patient is in heart block with a slow ventricular rate and the pacemaker fails to "sense" a QRS complex, it will discharge an electrical impulse and stimulate the heart. If the rate accelerates above a prescribed limit the pacemaker will automatically revert to standby as

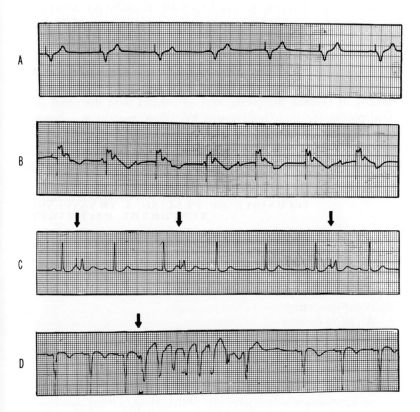

Fig. 7. Rhythm strips show pacemaker artefacts. A short "spike" precedes a wide QRS complex in A and B. A defective pacemaker discharges (arrow) on the vulnerable period of the T wave three times in lead C. In D the abnormally-timed pacemaker discharge produces a burst of ventricular tachycardia which spontaneously reverts back to sinus rhythm.

the "detected" QRS deactivates the power source momentarily. The demand type pacemaker is also equipped with variable voltage and variable rate. Demand pacing of heart has so many advantages there is no reason to use the fixed rate pacemaker any longer. Heart block due to myocardial infarction is transient. It may last from minutes to weeks. The demand pacemaker will function until the sinus node assumes the role of pacemaker. At that moment the pacemaker reverts to standby and eliminates the hazard of competition. Moreover, the demand pacemaker avoids the necessity of having to turn off the fixed rate pacemaker periodically to determine the inherent cardiac rhythm. Demand pacemakers have virtually no drawbacks, and are therefore highly desirable and used exclusively by us for heart block and sinus bradycardia in acute myocardial infarction.

Atrial pacing in patients with sinus rhythm offers a theoretic advantage because of the physiologic increase in cardiac output. Unfortunately, it does not work as well as desired due to the technical difficulty of keeping the pacing wire in contact with the atrial wall. Atrial pacing for sinus bradycardia has often resulted in secondary heart block when the atrial rate is accelerated, for the A-V node is incapable of tolerating rapid rates under certain circumstances. The only effective way to accelerate the heart rate is to pace the ventricles.

TECHNIQUE OF PLACING A TRANSVENOUS TEMPORARY PACEMAKER*

Before any attempt is made to introduce a transvenous pacemaker, several prophylactic measures should be taken and all equipment must be readily available. These include the following:

1. A defibrillator at the bedside.
2. A cut-down tray.
3. An ECG monitor.
4. Pacemaker wire.
5. Battery-powered pacemaker ("demand type").
6. Image intensifier. This makes the procedure infinitely easier, but a pacemaker can be introduced "blind" by trial and error when no fluoroscopic unit is available. Attempting to introduce a pacemaker blindly is recommended only in dire emergencies. There

---

* The authors as well as the physicians in the cardiac catheterization laboratory of St. Vincent's Hospital have been unsuccessful in "floating" the pacemaker wires into the ventricle, "blindly" or without fluoroscopy. We have abandoned this procedure and advocate the above technique.

is no risk in transporting the patient to an area where a fluoroscopic unit is available. At St. Vincent's Hospital this requires two elevator rides and a trip of two city blocks. There has been no morbidity from transporting patients. The patient should be monitored before any surgical manipulation is attempted. The defibrillator should be turned on and ready for use at the bedside.

Under xylocaine anesthesia with sterile technique the right external jugular vein is exposed and dissected free 1.0 cm above the clavicle. The antecubital vein may also be used but this approach is associated with more pacemaker failure owing to the tendency of the patients to move their arms. The right external jugular vein affords a direct course to the ventricle and leaves the left side free in case permanent pacemakers are necessary. Suture ligatures are placed proximally and distally on the exposed vein. Through a transverse incision a bipolar catheter pacemaker is inserted into the vein and advanced to the level of the right atrium. Care should be taken to keep the proximal ligature taut in order to prevent air embolus during inspiration.

Under fluoroscopy the catheter is advanced through the tricuspid valve so that its tip lies at the apex of the right ventricle (Fig. 8). This is probably the best location from which to pace the heart. The pacemaker is stable in this position and less likely to be dislodged by cardiac contraction, and cardiac perforation is least likely to occur in this position. The outflow tract of the right ventricle is the least suitable pacemaker site because of the instability of the catheter pacemaker. Moreover, it requires a greater degree of technical experience to place the pacemaker in the outflow tract. A common problem is that the pacemaker is inserted into the coronary sinus. Knowledge of fluoroscopic anatomy eliminates this difficulty. The ventricles can be paced from the coronary sinus but this is a poor place to leave the pacemaker catheter as it may tamponade venous return from the heart. Furthermore, it rarely stays in this site but dislodges and floats in the atrium.

Once the tip of the pacemaker wire is located at the apex of the right ventricle, an attempt may be made to pace the heart. The pacemaker wire is connected to the battery power with all settings turned to zero. The rate selector is adjusted first to a rate at least 10 to 15 beats per minute greater than the patient's own cardiac rate. Next the amperage is raised slowly while observing the oscilloscope. When the pacemaker deflection appears the ventricle is usually captured. If the ventricle fails to be captured at the first appearance of the pacemaker

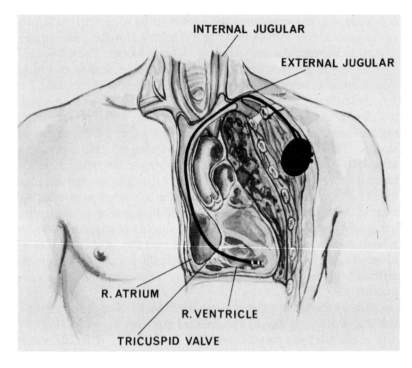

Fig. 8. A coronal diagram of the chest showing the placement of a pacemaker catheter in the apex of the right ventricle. This diagram shows a
permanent pacemaker battery placed subcutaneously. A temporary transvenous catheter is inserted in either the external jugular vein or the antecubital vein in a similar manner. (See text for description.)

deflection, the amperage is raised. Failure to capture the ventricles at
doses above two millivolts suggests either the rate selected is too slow
or, more likely, the pacemaker wire is not adjacent to the myocardium in which case appropriate steps may be taken. When pacing
begins the wire is firmly anchored to the vein with a suture ligature
and the wound is closed with interrupted sutures. Prophylactic antibiotics are prescribed so long as the pacemaker wire is in the heart.
Prostaphlin, one gram per day in divided dose, is effective.

HAZARDS OF TRANSVENOUS PACEMAKERS

1. While manipulating the catheter pacemaker in the heart, premature ventricular contractions may be produced. This is corrected

simply by withdrawing the catheter and repositioning it. After the pacemaker is in place and functioning, cardiosuppressive drugs (Quinidine) should be given until the pacemaker is removed.

2. Perforation of the myocardium: This is a rare but potentially serious complication. The catheter pacemaker should be removed immediately. A cardiocentesis tray is placed at the bedside and a thoracic or cardiac surgeon notified. Bleeding from a perforated myocardium may be scanty and require no therapy at all. If signs of pericardial effusion appear, pericardiocentesis is performed with aspiration of the blood. Surgery may be required to stop the bleeding. This must be very rare.

3. Competition: Isuprel is often prescribed while preparation is made to insert the pacemaker catheter. *Isuprel must be discontinued before any attempt is made to pace the heart*; otherwise ventricular tachycardia and fibrillation may ensue. The combination of adrenergic stimulation and external electrical stimulation produces marked ventricular irritability. Electrical competition between the patient's pacemaker and the electrical pacemaker may result in the electrical impulse falling on the T wave and may initiate ventricular fibrillation. The demand type pacemaker avoids this complication.

4. Failure to pace: The most common reason for pacemaker failure is movement of the tip of the pacemaker wire requiring some manipulation to restore it to a position adjacent to the myocardium. If the apex of the right ventricle is used this complication occurs less often than with other sites. Other causes of pacemaker failure include electrolyte derangements, especially hypokalemia. If serum potassium levels have been depleted by diuretics the administration of potassium salts orally or intravenously will correct this abnormality. The pacemaker may fail if the myocardium is perforated. A chest x-ray will usually confirm the diagnosis and therapy is simply to withdraw the catheter and proceed according to paragraph 2 above. Occasionally, a pacemaker will fail and require a progressive increase in amperage to maintain ventricular capture. The cause is not fully understood, but it is believed to be due to an ionic barrier that is built up around the tip of the pacemaker wire. If increasing the amperage does not correct the problem, replacement of the wire may be necessary.

The position of the electrode should be determined at least twice daily by turning up the cardiac rate and "capturing" the ventricle. This should be recorded on the ECG. The last check should be done before the "cath" lab closes for the day.

5. Broken wires: These are no longer a problem. Current manufacturing technology produces excellent long-lived wires.

6. Wires not connected to the battery box or shorting each other is one of the most common causes of pacing failure. Simple as it may seem the rush of inserting a pacemaker wire sometimes results in the improper connection of the pacemaker wire to the lead cable from the battery box. This should always be checked before manipulating the pacemaker catheter. More commonly the two external ends of the pacemaker wire are permitted to touch, thereby short-circuiting the battery current. The remedy consists of taping the brass connections to a tongue depressor and keeping the connections apart. If the patient is not being paced, first check the location of the pacemaker wires in relation to the power source.

7. Pericarditis. In approximately 10 percent of patients who have an intraventricular pacemaker wire (either permanent or temporary), a pericardial friction rub will develop. It is transient, lasting for a few hours to a few days. We have not altered the catheter pacemaker wire because of this and have seen no additional complication. It is not an indication for removal of the wire.

8. Sepsis. A shaking chill, fever and positive blood culture indicate infection in relation to the pacing wire. The fever may be septic or low grade. Fever is an indication for removal of the wire. Rarely has fever appeared before 10 days. In one patient we had to replace the wire in another vein, and this, together with changing the antibiotic, controlled the sepsis for a few days longer when sinus rhythm returned.

In an occasional patient electrical pacing through the right ventricle produces an alteration in the mechanical ejection from the heart with a resultant fall in cardiac output as opposed to maintaining or elevating the cardiac output. Although this happens infrequently it is necessary to be aware of it and discontinue the pacing promptly. This is shown in Figure 9.

DURATION OF TEMPORARY PACING

Rarely is it necessary to pace a patient for more than 4 days. One patient with complete heart block and slow ventricular pacemaker had to be paced for 11 days. The wire may be removed after 4 days, or 2 days after the need for it has disappeared.

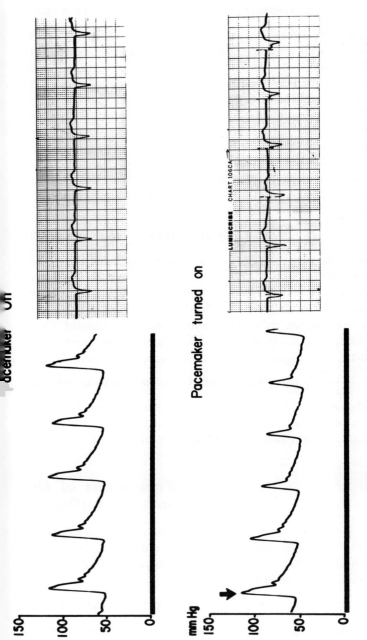

Fig. 9. An unusual effect of pacing the heart in acute myocardial infarct is graphically demonstrated. Blood pressure is 110/50 mm Hg during normal conduction. When the pacemaker is turned on (arrow) and the heart paced at an identical rate, the blood pressure falls to 70/50 mm Hg.

101

TRANSTHORACIC INTRACARDIAC PACEMAKER

Introducing a transvenous pacemaker during cardiac resuscitation is an extremely difficult and time-consuming procedure. The evolution of technique has led to a transthoracic intracardiac needle through which a fine pacemaker wire may be introduced through the chest wall and anchored to the endocardium somewhat like a fish hook. Experience with this procedure has not been satisfying and because the risk of pneumothorax is high, this procedure has been reserved for desperate situations—usually after cardiac arrest has occurred. For this and many other reasons the transvenous pacemaker should be introduced prophylactically. No survivors from cardiac arrest (asystole) have been seen in 15 consecutive attempts at transthoracic pacing.

EXTERNAL PACING (SKIN PACING)

During the early years of cardiac resuscitation, pacing the heart through paddles applied to the chest wall was commonly employed. We have never found this to be effective. While contraction of the pectoralis muscle is observed and sometimes an electrical ECG complex appears, effective pulse pressure has never been recorded. External cardiac pacing no longer has a place in the resuscitative armamentarium.

COUPLED PACING AND PAIRED PACING

Although such procedures can be done in patients, the clinical usefulness of the techniques is not established and the dangers not well defined. We have had no experience with this method.

Treatment of the Tachyarrhythmias

The tachyarrhythmias will be divided into two sections and we will first consider the supraventricular or atrial tachyarrhythmias: sinus tachycardia; APC (atrial premature contraction); atrial tachycardia; atrial flutter; atrial fibrillation.

SINUS TACHYCARDIA

Sinus tachycardia in acute myocardial infarction probably results from an attempt to raise cardiac output. Studies by Gorlin show that the infarcted myocardium fails to participate in ventricular systole due to an area of akinesis or dyskinesis.* Akinesis of the ventricular wall increases compliance, inhibits ventricular emptying, raises end diastolic pressure and lowers cardiac output. Dyskinesis of the ventricular wall allows the ventricular cavity to behave as if a ventricular aneurysm were present; thus, the radius of the ventricular sphere is increased resulting in increased work and oxygen consumption in a coronary system incapable of delivering adequate blood and oxygen. In both cases heart rate increases in an attempt to maintain cardiac output. The prognosis of sinus tachycardia is very serious because it indicates an extensive infarct.

Sinus tachycardia in acute myocardial infarction is sometimes unrelated to congestive heart failure, shock, or to lowered cardiac output. The most common causes under these circumstances are fever, hypovolemia secondary to bleeding stress ulcers, pulmonary embolus with or without pulmonary infarction, atelectasis, and infection.

Treatment is directed toward controlling systemic or precipitating factors. Fever associated with myocardial infarction may be elevated to very high levels (above 103 degrees). Salicylates are not always effective in reducing the temperature. The use of hypothermia blankets has not been systematically investigated but in isolated cases it has been found useful.

APPROACH TO THE PATIENT WITH SINUS TACHYCARDIA

Abnormalities in ventilation and oxygenation should be immediately corrected as should electrolyte derangements and acid-base disturbances. Hypovolemia may be corrected with the judicious replacement of volume expanders while constantly monitoring the central venous pressure. Pulmonary embolus should be treated with intravenous heparin unless a specific contraindication to its use exists.

Digitalis is usually not indicated in the treatment of sinus tachycardia without congestive heart failure. In desperate clinical circumstances it has been recommended. Ouabain is the digitalis preparation of choice because of its prompt onset of action and its rapid clearance which minimizes the hazard of toxicity. It is administered intravenously, 0.1 mg every 15 minutes, until an effect on the heart

---

* *Akinesis*: The infarcted muscle does not contract.
  Dyskinesis: The infarcted muscle bulges outward.

rate is noted or signs of toxicity—notably premature ventricular contractions—develop. The maximum dose is 0.5 mg in patients with acute myocardial infarction.

Recently, paired pulsing and coupled pulse pacing have been shown to be effective in controlling ventricular rates in sinus tachycardia. These methods have been tried in animal experiments and in non-infarcted human hearts. While ventricular rates have been controlled, no reduction in oxygen consumption or cardiac work has been demonstrated. It is unlikely that controlling sinus tachycardia by electrical means has any value in acute myocardial infarction. We have had no experience with these modalities.

Probably the best approach to the patient with marked sinus tachycardia is the same as that applied to the patient with unstable or very low blood pressure (see Shock). Monitoring of arterial and venous pressure, of urine flow, and arterial gas should be done and therapy should be directed by the findings based on the monitoring data.

ATRIAL PREMATURE CONTRACTION (APC)

Atrial premature contractions represent irritability of the atrial myocardium (Fig. 10). While atrial infarction is sometimes found at postmortem examinations, APC's are probably a manifestation of local ischemia due to involvement of the artery supplying the sinus node. APC's are less ominous than premature ventricular contractions. They rarely influence cardiac output or rate. When APC's appear repetitively they may herald the onset of atrial flutter or atrial fibrillation. Isolated APC's are usually not treated. When APC's appear in bigeminy or repetitively (more than 10 per minute), they

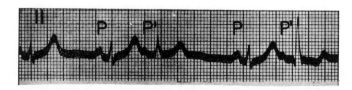

Fig. 10.　Rhythm strip demonstrating atrial premature contraction. The appearance of atrial premature contractions denote hypoxemia and often herald the onset of atrial fibrillation. (From Kennedy, Grace, and Flood. *Medical Resident's Manual*, 2nd Ed., 1966. Courtesy of Appleton-Century-Crofts.)

should be controlled. Treatment starts with adequate ventilation and oxygenation. Quinidine is next prescribed starting with 200 mg every 6 hours by mouth. More vigorous therapy (400 mg) is usually not necessary for control.

ATRIAL TACHYCARDIA, ATRIAL FLUTTER AND ATRIAL FIBRILLATION (THE SUPRAVENTRICULAR TACHYARRHYTHMIAS)

The supraventricular tachyarrhythmias, atrial tachycardia, flutter, and fibrillation, having similar effects on coronary circulation, are grouped together. These in common represent atrial ectopic activity with varying degrees of ventricular response. The net result is a rapid ventricular rate producing failing circulation.

Coronary blood flow is directly dependent on aortic pulse pressure. With rapid supraventricular arrhythmias, cardiac output and central aortic pressure fall, thus compromising coronary circulation. It is estimated that coronary perfusion falls an average of 35 percent during episodes of tachycardia. Ventricular tachycardia decreases coronary circulation by as much as 60 percent. Thus, bouts of rapid heart action in myocardial infarction are self-defeating since the fall-off in coronary circulation further aggravates hypoxia of the myocardium. The ectopic tachyarrhythmias are also similar in that their appearance may be brief and reversion to normal rhythm spontaneous. Unfortunately, it is not possible to know which will cease spontaneously. Recognition of the arrhythmia is indication enough to institute positive steps toward treatment. The ectopic focus responds to adequate ventilation and antiarrhythmic drugs. When myocardial infarction is healed sinus rhythm is usually maintained.

It is probable that ectopic atrial rhythms are well tolerated by the coronary patient as long as the ventricular rate remains between 60 and 120; otherwise, tachyarrhythmias must be promptly controlled because they reduce central aortic blood pressure. The healthy patient can tolerate any one of the supraventricular tachyarrhythmias for prolonged periods. In the setting of myocardial infarction they represent a catastrophe, for the reduced cardiac output in tachycardia compromises the already-compromised coronary circulation (Fig. 11).

Given a patient with a sinus mechanism who suffers a myocardial infarct and then suddenly develops a supraventricular tachyarrhythmia—what should be done? Adequate ventilation should be instituted and any derangements of acid-base balance corrected. Next

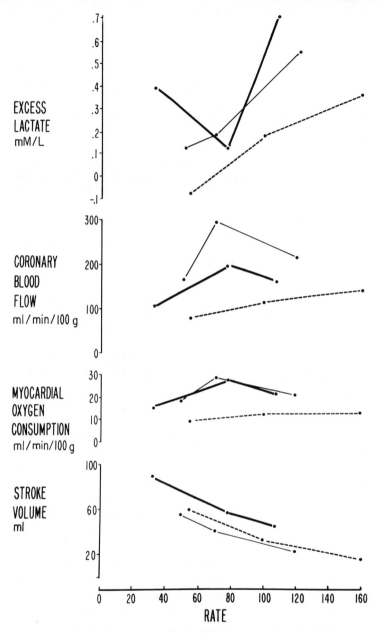

Fig. 11. The relationship between heart rate and myocardial energetics in three patients. Increasing heart rate decreases stroke volume, produces an inconstant change in coronary blood flow and oxygen consumption, and markedly increases the production of excess lactate indicating the development of anaerobic metabolism. Each patient is indicated by a different type of line. (Adapted from Ayres and Giannelli. *Care of the Critically Ill*, 1967. Courtesy of Appleton-Century-Crofts.)

quinidine should be prescribed. In our patients with acute myocardial infarction, quinidine converted as many as 50 percent of cases. The remainder had to be cardioverted electrically 4 hours after the last meal using Valium anesthesia (see p. 89). Quinidine will maintain the conversion by suppression of the ectopic focus. If quinidine is not prescribed before cardioversion, the relapse rate is high.

The usual premedicating dose of quinidine is 400 mg given intramuscularly about 1 hour before the conversion is attempted. Accelerated conduction is rarely encountered. Should accelerated conduction ensue, such as 1:1 conduction with atrial flutter, then electric conversion is carried out immediately. Maintenance therapy of 200 mg of quinidine by mouth every 6 hours is prescribed for as long as 7 to 10 days. As a rule, prolonged quinidine therapy is not prescribed since ectopic tachyarrhythmias are usually due to transient ischemia. Once infarction heals, sinus rhythm returns, and quinidine should be discontinued. If the patient reverts to an ectopic atrial arrhythmia, additional therapy with quinidine must be given.

A problem arises in the patient with chronic atrial fibrillation who suffers an infarct or the patient with an infarct who presents with atrial fibrillation of an undetermined or unknown duration. Conversion of chronic atrial fibrillation may be hazardous owing to the high incidence of systemic embolization. To subject a patient to the hazard of drug or electric conversion under these circumstances is unwarranted. Cardioversion is avoided and digitalis may be used with caution to control the ventricular rate.

ATRIAL TACHYCARDIAS WITH RAPID VENTRICULAR RATE

This arrhythmia is infrequently found in acute myocardial infarct, but when it is detected it is commonly associated with anterior wall infarction. Direct current countershock is the treatment of choice. A case record will serve to illustrate this point.

CASE REPORT:

A 56-year-old man with chest pain came to the Emergency Room of St. Vincent's Hospital. He had had a myocardial infarction 2 years previously, but otherwise was well and asymptomatic until one half-hour before admission. An electrocardiogram showed atrial tachycardia of 180 per minute. Q waves were present in L2, L3 and AVF, with ST segment depression in the lateral precordial leads. During the examination the patient complained of excruciating crushing anterior chest pain. The blood pressure began to fall and the patient started to thrash about in bed. Direct current countershock was instituted, with immediate reversion of the arrhythmia to sinus rhythm at a rate of 100 per minute. Chest pain ceased. During the subsequent days an anterior wall infarction evolved, from which the patient recovered.

Had there been any further delay in the control of this arrhythmia, it is doubtful that the patient would have survived. Drug therapy will probably have taken too long to work. Carotid sinus pressure, Valsalva maneuvers, and other vagal stimulators usually used for atrial tachycardia unassociated with infarction are of little value, although they may be tried while preparation is being made to convert the arrhythmia electrically.

ATRIAL TACHYCARDIA WITH BLOCK

Atrial tachycardia with block, manifesting digitalis toxicity in acute infarction, is distinctly uncommon (Fig. 12). Occasionally, a patient taking digitalis, undergoing vigorous diuresis with marked kaliuresis, may develop PAT with block. In these cases the treatment is obviously potassium replacement. The differential between digitalis-induced atrial tachycardia with block and atrial flutter is often difficult. The differentiation is important as electric cardioversion in flutter is safe and effective, whereas it is likely to be dangerous in digitalis-induced atrial tachycardia. The following points may help in the differentiation:

	ATRIAL RATE	VENT. RATE	VENT. RHYTHM	BASE LINE OF ATRIAL WAVES	CHANCE OF DIGITALIS INTOXICATION
Atrial tachycardia with block (digitalis)	150 (240 or less)	120 or less	usually irregular	base is isoelectric	high
Atrial flutter (no digitalis)	240+ usually 300	150	usually regular	undulating base line	low

In cases of real urgency electric cardioversion may be attempted, but very low energy levels must be used. Lown recommends levels as low as 5 watt-seconds in arrhythmia due to digitalis.

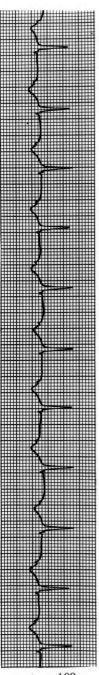

Fig. 12. Rhythm strip demonstrating atrial tachycardia with block due to digitalis toxicity. The atrial rate is 166 beats and the ventricular rate 83 beats per minute. The arrhythmia was recorded from a patient who was taking digoxin, 0.25 mgm daily for atrial fibrillation who then sustained a transmural myocardial infarction and received potent diuretics without potassium replacement. Replacement of potassium salts and the temporary discontinuation of digitalis resulted in a reversion to atrial fibrillation.

If the atrial arrhythmia is digitalis-induced, electrical cardioversion in low dosage will result in numerous APC's, atrial fibrillation, or at least acceleration of the atrial rate. If the electrical energy administered is low, these arrhythmias are short-lived and generally not dangerous. If the electrical energy is large, such arrhythmias may progress and be fatal. If the electric cardioversion is followed by the above arrhythmias indicating that the arrhythmia is digitalis-induced, electric cardioversion must be abandoned and drug treatment with quinidine or propanolol instituted.

SUMMARY (ATRIAL TACHYCARDIA)

Diagnosis: Rate of 180 to 220/minute with each ventricular complex preceded by a P wave.
Treatment: Direct current countershock. Ancillary measures: 1) adequate oxygenation of the patient; 2) quinidine gluconate, 400 mg, I.M.; 3) elevate blood pressure with small doses of aramine; 4) Pronestyl I.V., 500 mg in 500 cc D/W, until an effect is noted.

Atrial tachycardia with block due to digitalis. *Treatment*: Withhold digitalis, treat with potassium or propanolol. Use electric cardioversion only in dire emergency and start with low electrical energy levels.

ATRIAL FLUTTER

Atrial flutter is considered to be a rare arrhythmia during acute myocardial infarction (Fig. 13). Our experience during the past 4 years has been quite the opposite. We encounter atrial flutter six times in the course of 100 myocardial infarctions. The patients present a remarkably similar picture in that they generally have anterior wall infarction and have ventricular rates between 140 and 150 beats per minute. The regularity of the ventricular rate has allowed us to establish a dictum that "pulse rates of 150/minute are due to atrial flutter until proven otherwise." This arrhythmia is easily confused with sinus tachycardia. Such an error is not permissible because 1) the treatment of atrial flutter is simple, and 2) after treatment is instituted, ventricular rates under 100/minute can be maintained.

The treatment of atrial flutter in acute myocardial infarction is electric cardioversion, which is usually successful. Once the electrocardiographic diagnosis of atrial flutter is made and confirmed, the patient is given 400 mg of quinidine gluconate intramuscularly. He is

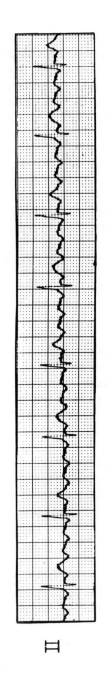

II

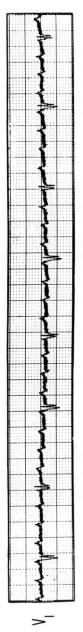

V₁

Fig. 13. Atrial flutter with a high degree of A-V block is shown. The ventricular rate is approximately 72 beats per minute. Cardioversion is not indicated as long as the ventricular rate remains between 60 and 100 beats per minute and the blood pressure is normal.

111

then to have nothing by mouth. Under the effect of large doses of quinidine, about half the patients revert spontaneously to sinus rhythm and do not need the electric cardioversion. Four hours after the last meal, electric cardioversion is performed under light general amnesia. Of the group who do not convert with quinidine alone, 90 percent convert with electric cardioversion following which the patient is given a maintenance dose of quinidine by mouth every 6 hours for one week. If no premature atrial contractions are seen, quinidine may be discontinued. If premature atrial contractions appear regularly, then quinidine is continued until such time as their appearance is sporadic. Previous objection to this mode of therapy rested in the time-honored custom of controlling the ventricles with digitalis before converting the patient, lest a 1:1 conduction ensue and produce ventricular rates above 200. We have seen this happen only once. If it does occur and the ventricular rate is too rapid, cardioversion should be performed at once.

SUMMARY

Diagnosis: Atrial rate 280-320 per minute;
              Ventricular rate 140-160—usual;
              2:1 conduction most common;
              4:1 and 3:1 conduction less common.

Treatment: Quinidine gluconate, 400 mg, I.M.;
              N.P.O.;
              Cardiovert after 4 hours under light general amnesia (use Valium);
              Maintenance quinidine, 200 mg, every 6 hours, p.o., for 1 week or more.

ATRIAL FIBRILLATION

Approximately 10 percent of patients with myocardial infarction develop acute atrial fibrillation (Fig. 14). Some patients were having atrial fibrillation before the infarction. Patients who have atrial fibrillation with acute infarction usually have rapid ventricular rates. Often this is associated with congestive heart failure. Prompt therapy is mandatory. In patients with acute fibrillation, controlling the ventricular

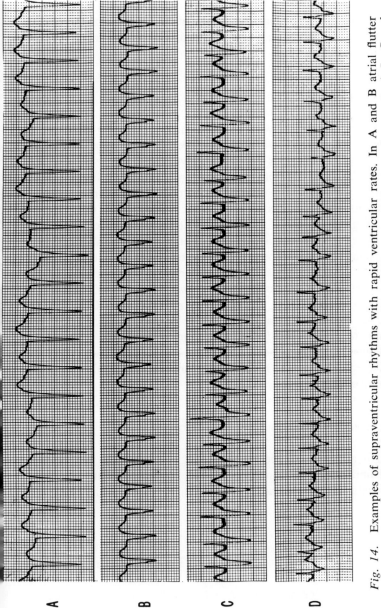

Fig. 14. Examples of supraventricular rhythms with rapid ventricular rates. In A and B atrial flutter with 2:1 A-V block and ventricular rates in excess of 150 beats per minute are demonstrated. In C and D atrial fibrillation with rapid ventricular rates are shown. See text for description of treatment.

rate sometimes cures the congestive failure. In patients with chronic atrial fibrillation and congestive heart failure, digitalis is required. For the purpose of discussion we have categorized the most common clinical situations.

Atrial Fibrillation of Recent Onset

When the patient with an acute myocardial infarction who is known to have been in sinus rhythm presents with atrial fibrillation, the treatment of choice is electric cardioversion, if the ventricular rate is over 120. Reestablishing sinus rhythm is important because regular atrial contraction may add 25 percent to the cardiac output. Treatment is the same as for atrial flutter. The patient, fully oxygenated, is given quinidine and later electrically cardioverted. Giving large doses of quinidine in atrial fibrillation results in about 50 percent reverting spontaneously. Of the remainder, about 50 percent more will revert to sinus rhythm with electric cardioversion. If the patient cannot be cardioverted after two doses of 400 joules, the procedure is abandoned. If ventricular rates above 120 per minute continue, digitalis is usually prescribed. Ventricular rates below 110 per minute are not considered harmful unless associated with congestive failure. Digitalis is not prescribed for atrial fibrillation with ventricular rates below 120 per minute unless associated with frank congestive heart failure.

Atrial Fibrillation of Long Duration

No attempt is made to cardiovert a patient who has been in atrial fibrillation for more than a year. If such a patient sustains a myocardial infarct the rapid arrhythmia is treated with digitalis.

Ventricular Tachyarrhythmias

The following will now be considered: ventricular premature contraction (VPC); ventricular flutter and fibrillation; ventricular tachycardia.

VENTRICULAR PREMATURE CONTRACTION (VPC)

Ventricular premature contraction is the most common arrhythmia encountered in myocardial infarctions. In most large series the incidence is about 80 percent. The mechanism of VPC is not completely known. One group considers VPC's to represent a re-entry phenomenon in the atrioventricular junctional tissue. Another favors the theory of an irritable focus which exists at the border between ischemic and normal myocardium. The general indications for the treatment of VPC are the following and is the system used by us.

1. VPC's with a frequency of 5 or more per minute (more than one per sweep of the monitor screen).
2. VPC's which appear in salvos of two or more in sequence.
3. VPC's which encroach or fall upon the downstroke of the preceding T wave (the R on T phenomenon), the so-called vulnerable period.

The following diagram (Fig. 15) shows this relationship as do the ECG's shown in Figure 16.

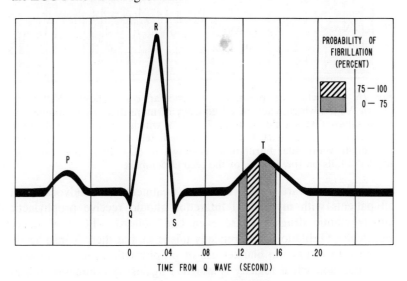

Fig. 15. A schematic diagram of the vulnerable period of the T wave. If a premature ventricular contraction falls within the cross-hatched area, the probability of producing ventricular fibrillation is 75 to 100 percent. Premature ventricular contractions falling in the shaded area have a probability of inducing ventricular fibrillation of 0 to 75 percent. (Adapted from Lown. *Sci. Amer.*, 219:19, 1968).

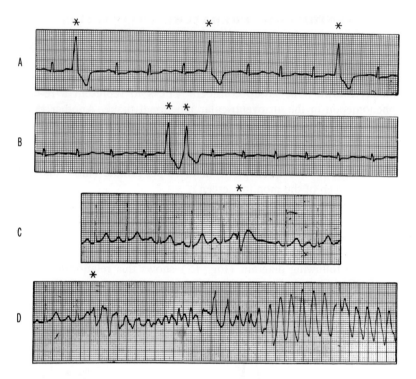

Fig. 16. Varieties of premature ventricular contractions (VPC) are shown. VPC's which occur in a frequency of more than 5 per minute (A) or in salvos (B) should be treated. VPC's which fall on the vulnerable period of the T wave (C) must be immediately treated since they may precipitate ventricular fibrillation, as shown in (D). In strip D note that the VPC falls on the T wave of the second complex.

Isolated or rare VPC's require no treatment. Some advocate that all patients with myocardial infarction should receive prophylactic antiarrhythmic drugs because even one isolated VPC can induce ventricular fibrillation. Theoretically this is so, but there is insufficient evidence to justify the blanket use of prophylactic drugs in myocardial infarction when toxicity is weighed against questionable indications.

Therapy of premature ventricular contractions includes the following:

1. Maintenance of adequate oxygenation. Hypoxemia alone may propogate VPC's.

CASE REPORT:

A 48-year-old man had recurrent bouts of premature ventricular contraction uncontrolled by xylocaine, quinidine and procainamide. Extreme irritability was attributed to cerebral hypoxemia and falling cardiac output. In the process of being intubated to improve ventilation his artificial teeth were found lodged in his larynx. When the teeth were removed ventilation improved and all VPC's disappeared.

We emphasize that the patient's color is not a reliable index of oxygenation. If VPC's appear repetitively, arterial oxygen tension should be determined and appropriate steps taken to correct existing abnormalities.

2. Maintenance of normal pH. The most arrhythmogenic abnormality is alkalosis. Myocardial infarction induces alkalosis because of hypoxemia which develops and leads to hyperventilation. Correction of alkalosis includes the administration of oxygen and control of ventilation if necessary. (See Chapter 4)

3. Drug therapy is effective in controlling VPC's. The drug of choice is Lidocaine (xylocaine without epinephrine) intravenously, administered as a bolus of 25 mg I.V., followed if necessary in 2 minutes by an additional 25 mg. A Lidocaine drip may be started at a dose of from 1 to 4 mg per minute and may be continued for 48 hours if necessary. No more than 2,000 mg per 24 hours should be given. Rare idiosyncrasy to the drug is manifested by convulsions. The seizures are treated by discontinuing the drug and administering Valium 5-10 mg I.V. Lidocaine is a superior drug in the treatment of VPC's because its prompt action brings results in a few minutes. Next in order of effectiveness is quinidine given orally or intramuscularly in a dose of 200 mg every 6 hours. This dose may be increased to 400 or 600 mg if necessary, but with increasing doses toxicity may appear. Idiosyncrasies to quinidine manifested by syncope and respiratory and cardiac arrest and ventricular fibrillation are rare. In the past year, we have seen two such patients. Recurrent ventricular fibrillation in a patient receiving quinidine or procainamide should raise the question of quinidine toxicity. Intravenous molar lactate is said to be of some use in reversing this complication. Procainamide has no advantage over quinidine in antiarrhythmic effect except that in addition to oral use it may be prescribed by vein. It is useful as maintenance therapy after intravenous xylocaine has been prescribed for several days. The

usual dose is one gram every 6 hours by mouth. Fifteen grams per day have been given with no serious complications.

Should premature ventricular contractions fail to respond to this regimen, complicating factors such as congestive heart failure and bradycardia must be considered. VPC's may be a sign of diminishing cardiac output in the course of congestive heart failure. Therapy is then directed to increasing cardiac output and improving oxygenation by employing digitalis and diuretics. Antiarrhythmic agents are contraindicated when premature contractions are caused by congestive failure. VPC's may appear as escape beats during bradyarrhythmia. Under these conditions cardiac depressive drugs are not used. If the ventricles are accelerated the VPC's disappear. Therapy may include atropine for sinus bradycardia or transvenous electric pacemakers for refractory sinus bradycardia, nodal rhythm and heart block with slow ventricular rates.

Ventricular premature contractions as manifestation of digitalis excess should be readily diagnosed. The treatment is to discontinue the digitalis. Intravenous Dilantin, 250 mg in one bolus, may also be included.

VENTRICULAR FIBRILLATION

The following experience with ventricular fibrillation is from our own Coronary Care Unit and Emergency Room.

Total patients (consecutive transmural myocardial infarction)		625
Patients with primary ventricular fibrillation		85
In Coronary Care Unit	44	
In Emergency Room	32	
	76	
In General Hospital	9	
Percent Overall Survivors		68%
Percent survivors in Coronary Care Unit	41%	
Percent survivors in Emergency Room	75%	

Approximately 75 percent of the patients we see with acute myocardial infarction enter the Emergency Room within 4 hours of the onset of the severe pain. This probably accounts for the relatively large number of patients seen with ventricular fibrillation. If a hospital is receiving patients 8 to 10 hours after the onset of pain, less ventricular fibrillation will be encountered because many patients with this arrhythmia will have already died.

Ventricular fibrillation occurs at any time of the day or night or in any month. We felt at one time that the patients did not have ventricular fibrillation except during the "working" hours of the Coronary Care Unit (9:00 A.M. to 9:00 P.M.) and that once the patient was asleep ventricular fibrillation no longer appeared. Continued experience may not bear this out but at present we feel that ventricular fibrillation does not often occur in the *sleeping* patient.

Monthly statistics for ventricular fibrillation show no variations as shown in the following consecutive attempts at resuscitation for ventricular fibrillation in acute myocardial infarction.

SEASONAL VARIATION IN VENTRICULAR FIBRILLATION

	ALIVE	DEAD
January	0	0
February	2	1
March	3	5
April	1	3
May	1	0
June	0	1
July	1	2
August	4	1
September	3	1
October	2	1
November	1	1
December	0	1
	18	17

The variations from month to month are probably not significant.

VENTRICULAR FIBRILLATION: TREATMENT

Ventricular fibrillation is the hub about which all discussion of resuscitation is centered. For this life-terminating arrhythmia almost nothing that can be done which will make the situation worse. Ventricular fibrillation is frequently heralded by premonitory warning arrhythmias such as ventricular premature beats or bursts of ventricular tachycardia. In some cases and especially on the first hospital day of myocardial infarction, there may be no warning. *Primary ventricular fibrillation* is ventricular fibrillation in the absence of shock or heart failure Secondary ventricular fibrillation is the terminal event of complicating diseases such as severe cardiac failure and shock. The patient with ventricular fibrillation due to acute myocardial infarction is dead unless something is done to restore his circulation. At the present time, there is only one effective treatment and that is defibrillation using electric current. No effective drug is available. Bretylium tosylate (300 mg I.M.), an experimental drug, shows much promise but at the present time is still in the developmental phase.

Prevention of ventricular fibrillation is of prime importance. Ventricular premature beats and ventricular tachycardia must be effectively suppressed. Hypoxia and acidosis must be corrected. While some physicians claim the complete prevention of primary ventricular fibrillation in the Coronary Care Unit, others feel that this arrhythmia may occasionally appear in the otherwise stable patient with acute myocardial infarction. Especially on the first hospital day, more than at any other time, one must be keenly alert for the occurrence of ventricular fibrillation. Sudden and unexpected ventricular fibrillation may occur at any time for about 14 days after admission but is less frequent with the passing of each day.

The essence of the treatment of ventricular fibrillation is prompt action. The longer fibrillation continues the more profound will be the acidosis which of itself interferes with and prevents restoration of normal rhythm. The following table outlines the difficulty which is encountered with delayed action and indicates the magnitude of the dose of bicarbonate required to correct the acidosis.

PATIENT	MINUTES AFTER ARREST	pH	P_{CO_2}	EKG	TREATMENT
1	30	7.10	56	V. Fib.	
	60	7.26	42	V. Fib.	100 mEq HCO_3
2	5	7.00	60	V. Fib.	
	30	7.34	45	S. R.	400 mEq HCO_3
3	10	7.25	36	V. Fib.	
	25	7.36	42	V. Fib.-S. R.	200 mEq HCO_3
	55	7.38	47	S. R.	200 mEq HCO_3
4	35	7.08	48	V. Fib.	100 mEq HCO_3
	50	7.30	39	S. R.	100 mEq HCO_3
	24 hours	7.45	38	S. R.	

Note that large doses of bicarbonate must be given. For example, 400 mEq or 8 ampules of the usually available material.

From Thomson W.S.T.: In Shaw, G., ed. Resuscitation and Cardiac Pacing. Philadelphia, F. A. Davis, 1965, p. 69.

Although one can maintain some cardiac output in ventricular fibrillation with closed chest cardiac massage, the longer the patient has an inadequate cardiac output, the more severe will be his hypoxia and metabolic acidosis. The first order of importance is to defibrillate the heart and only then start cardiac massage and ventilation. If cardiac massage and artificial ventilation are carried out for more than a few minutes, the ensuing acidosis must be corrected with intravenous sodium bicarbonate for the acidotic patient is very resistant to defibrillation. After a loading dose of 88 mEq of sodium bicarbonate, 44 mEq should be given every 10 minutes for as long as resuscitation continues. Attempting to administer 44 mEq (50 cc) repeatedly is time-consuming. For this reason an intravenous injection of 5 percent $NaHCO_3$ solution should be continuously administered until circulation is restored.

Several factors delay or interfere with successful defibrillation. The *first* is inertia. The following tabulation derived from animal laboratory teaching experiences clearly indicates the importance of having the equipment in meticulous order and the team fully experienced (see also p. 86).

TIME REQUIRED TO DEFIBRILLATE (EXPERIMENTAL ANIMAL OR MANIKIN)

30 seconds	Shortest possible time
65 seconds	Could not get the cap off the jelly tube
90 seconds	Could not find the electrical socket
2 minutes +	No jelly on the cart
65 seconds	Pushed wrong switch
75 seconds	Too many wires in the drawer

The *second factor* is resistance of the fibrillatory waves to countershock. If ventricular fibrillation is inadvertently allowed to persist, the fibrillatory waves become "fine" or almost imperceptible on the surface electrocardiogram and experience has shown that fine fibrillation is resistant to countershock. Epinephrine, 1 cc of 1:1,000 diluted in 10 cc of water injected directly into the cardiac chamber through the chest wall, may make "fine" fibrillatory waves "coarse" and susceptible to defibrillation. The technic of injecting intracardiac epinephrine is not as simple as it may seem. The cardiac needle is placed in the fifth intercostal space to the left of the sternum and directed medial and cephalad with constant aspiration of the barrel of the syringe. When the ventricular cavity is entered a prompt return of blood is seen. The contents of the syringe are quickly injected and external cardiac massage is again instituted in an effort to deliver the epinephrine to the left ventricular myocardium. Precious time is often wasted in making this injection which could be devoted to proper oxygenation and correction of acidosis. Closed chest massage and pulmonary ventilation must not be interrupted during this maneuver.

The *third factor* preventing defibrillation is hypoxia. If defibrillation is instituted within one minute of ventricular fibrillation, assisted ventilation with an Ambu bag is all that is necessary. If there is delay in defibrillation and the heart is refractory to defibrillation, endotracheal intubation will be necessary with controlled ventilation until hypoxia is corrected. During intubation and ventilation, closed-chest cardiac massage must be vigorously continued. Once spontaneous circulation is restored, the patient may regain consciousness. However, this is not always so and patients have remained in coma for as long as 48 hours and, ultimately, made a complete recovery There has *never* been a long-term decerebrate survivor in over 625 cases of acute myocardial infarction and only one in many thousands of attempted resuscitations for other disorders. To reemphasize, the patient with ventricular fibrillation is dead unless something is done promptly. On this basis nurses have been taught to do closed-chest cardiac massage and institute immediate defibrillation. There may be medico-legal implications against permitting nurses to perform this necessary procedure. Where nurses are allowed to perform this very vital treatment, little harm has been done. Inasmuch as without treatment death is the outcome, what harm can be done?

Ventricular Fibrillation and Complete Heart Block

Ventricular fibrillation in the presence of complete heart block is due to bradycardia and falling cardiac output. Consequently antiarrhythmic, cardiodepressant medication is contraindicated in A-V block. Procainamide and quinidine should not be used lest fibrillation recur. The treatment of ventricular fibrillation in patients with complete heart block consists of electric defibrillation as above and acceleration of the ventricular rate. This is accomplished by a transvenous temporary pacemaker. While it takes time to insert a pacemaker, isoproterenol may be given as an intravenous drip to accelerate ventricular rate. One ampule is diluted in 250 cc of dextrose solution and titrated until a ventricular rate of 60/minute is restored.

Extreme care must be exercised to discontinue isoproterenol before turning on a pacemaker so as not to induce irreversible ventricular fibrillation.

VENTRICULAR TACHYCARDIA

Experience from cardiac monitoring indicates that ventricular tachycardia may be paroxysmal or sustained (Fig. 17). Ventricular tachycardia will not sustain the circulation and will result in ventricular fibrillation. Only rarely does prolonged sustained tachycardia cease spontaneously. According to one study, ventricular tachycardia, or more than three successive ventricular ectopic beats, appeared in 99 of 300 monitored patients with acute myocardial infarction.

The treatment of paroxysmal ventricular tachycardia is intravenous xylocaine. A bolus of 50 mg injected intravenously may be repeated in 30 minutes if necessary. A continuous drip of 1 gram in a liter of dextrose solution per 24 hours is instituted. Less may be used if ventricular ectopic beats are suppressed. More than 2 grams per 24 hours is dangerous owing to cerebral toxicity with convulsions. If increasing doses of xylocaine are required, it may be necessary to employ procainamide, 250 mg, or quinidine, 200 mg, every 6 hours. Very large doses are sometimes necessary and as much as 15 grams of procainamide per day have been used without deleterious results. Sustained ventricular tachycardia should be promptly cardioverted. Direct current countershock may be delivered more promptly than drugs. Whichever treatment can be delivered most quickly should be used. Anesthesia is unnecessary under such circumstances because cardiac output and blood pressure are falling and the patient is in dire condition. Once conversion is carried out, xylocaine should be administered intravenously as a prophylactic. Recurrent ventricular tachycardia is considered a major change in the patient's condition and the entire CCU must be mobilized (see Chapter 9, p. 190).

Bretylium Tosylate

Bretylium tosylate has been found to raise the ventricular fibrillation threshold to electrical current. In clinical medicine it has been used in doses of 100 mg given slowly intravenously and 300 mg intramuscularly. The ECG diagnosis of ventricular tachycardia is especially difficult. Supraventricular tachycardia with aberrant conduction

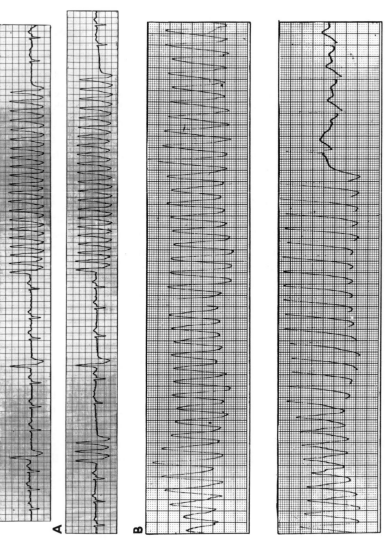

Fig. 17. Paroxysmal ventricular tachycardia (A) is characterized by bursts of three or more ventricular contractions in sequence. Note the frequency of isolated premature ventricular beats. Sustained ventricular tachycardia is unable to support the circulation and almost always terminates in ventricular fibrillation. Ventricular tachycardia spontaneously reverts to sinus rhythm, an exception to the rule. Ven-

is much more common than ventricular tachycardia. Ventricular tachycardia does not maintain the circulation. Supraventricular tachycardia will sustain circulation for a considerable time. The importance of oxygen for these patients cannot be overemphasized. Patients with recurrent arrhythmias are probably hypoxic and prompt attention must be given to this factor.

Bradyarrhythmia and Block

Bradyarrhythmia means slow ventricular rate (pulse or QSR rate below 50). Because first degree heart block and second degree heart block may lead to third degree heart block, they are included in the bradyarrhythmias. Because bundle branch block (BBB) may herald the appearance of third degree heart block, it is included in this section.

Patients with inferior and inferoposterior infarction are subject to bradyarrhythmia more than those with anterior infarction. Given a patient with inferior infarct, one must be alert to the possible appearance of the slow heart rate syndromes. The A-V node is supplied by the right coronary in 85 percent of patients.

There are many conflicting estimates of the frequency of the bradyarrhythmias. Data prior to continuous monitoring probably represent only selected cases. Even in the era of continuous monitoring there are wide ranges of the reported incidence. From the studies of Dr. J. F. Pantridge it has become apparent that bradyarrhythmia is an early event in acute myocardial infarction. Hence, as pointed out above (Chapter 1, p. 11), in order to compare one series with another, one must know the hour or day in the life history of the infarction. Until this is done no statistics of incidence are reliable and no two series may be compared. In our own series of patients who were seen from 4 to 6 hours after onset of pain, the following incidence of bradyarrhythmia was seen:

INCIDENCE OF BRADYARRHYTHMIA IN ACUTE INFARCTION:
ST. VINCENT'S HOSPITAL

Sinus Bradycardia	12.5%
1° Heart Block	10.2%
2° Heart Block	4.9%
3° Heart Block	7.0%
Junctional Rhythm	4.2%

Our own experience, as well as that of Pantridge, suggests that the bradyarrhythmias and A-V block seen earlier—i.e., the first hospital day—are of greater threat to life than those that occur in the 3rd or 4th hospital day.

HEMODYNAMIC ASPECTS OF SLOW HEART RATE

As the ventricular rate slows, the cardiac output falls in a straight line relationship. However, when the heart rate goes below 40 to 50, the fall in cardiac output is precipitous. The available data in patients with acute infarction is scanty. However, it is generally felt that the fall-off in output at slow ventricular rates represents more than can be attributed to the slow rate alone. As indicated in other sections the perfusion of the coronary arteries is proportional to central aortic pressure. There is probably an optimal central pressure for coronary perfusion. There is certainly a critical perfusion pressure around 60 mm mean aortic pressure. Perfusion pressure falls off at slow heart rates As the perfusion pressure falls, oxygenation of the myocardium becomes further reduced, cardiac output is further diminished, and a vicious cycle is established. The end result may be an Adams-Stokes attack or ventricular fibrillation. Too much emphasis should not be placed on knowing the cardiac output at various heart rates. Attempts to establish treatment regimens for the problem of heart block and sinus bradycardia based solely on the cardiac output data seem to us to avoid one of the main problems. *The electric pacemaker can prevent Adams-Stokes attacks and for this reason may be life-saving.*

As indicated, the causes of death in the monitored patients are as follows:

Ventricular fibrillation	12%
Asystole	20%
Shock	30%
Heart failure	10%

Asystole accounts for 20 percent of our deaths. We *assume* that much of this asystole is heralded by bradyarrhythmia and bundle branch blocks. We *advocate* early placing of the electric pacemaker in the bradyarrhythmic states. To state the situation in another way: besides the obvious hazard of low cardiac output with slow heart rates, a serious consequence of bradyarrhythmias is electric instability. Asystole and death may ensue from any bradyarrhythmia or heart block. Asystole may also result from a progressive sinus bradycardia. Ectopic or "escape" ventricular tachyarrhythmias may arise from slow heart rates of any cause but especially heart block. This is often a cause of Adams-Stokes attacks in both chronic and acute heart block. There appears to be a critically slow heart rate below which the appearance of escape ventricular tachyarrhythmias are more prone to occur. This critical rate is generally below 40 beats per minute. First and second degree heart block are hazardous only in that they may progress to complete heart block. Second degree block is particularly dangerous because a high degree of block may follow resulting in a very slow ventricular rate. Such degrees of block are an adequate warning of electrical and conductive instability and should be heeded.

SUMMARY

Bradyarrhythmias are considered dangerous in themselves. They are considered an early warning sign of impending disaster. Faced with one of the bradyarrhythmias (sinus bradyarrhythmia, heart block, junctional rhythms) one must make two separate decisons:

1. On the diagnosis of the bradyarrhythmia or heart block (second or third degree) or certain instances of bundle branch block, the electric pacemaker must be placed regardless of the present ventricular rate.

2. If the ventricular rate is below 50, the electricity should be turned on and the ventricle paced at 65 to 70 beats/minute.

The use of the demand pacemaker obviates much of the decision making in 2. The demand pacemaker is adjusted to activate at rates below 65.

Placing the electric pacemaker is not as simple as it sounds; it should be done while the hospital is "awake" (during the hours of 9 A.M. to 5 P.M.) and done promptly. Once the end of the working day comes it will take 2 to 3 hours to get the pacemaker in place. Because of our high mortality in elderly persons and in persons with bundle branch block (see below), we suggest that the following clinical situations be used to alert the staff promptly to the possibility of a pacemaker insertion:

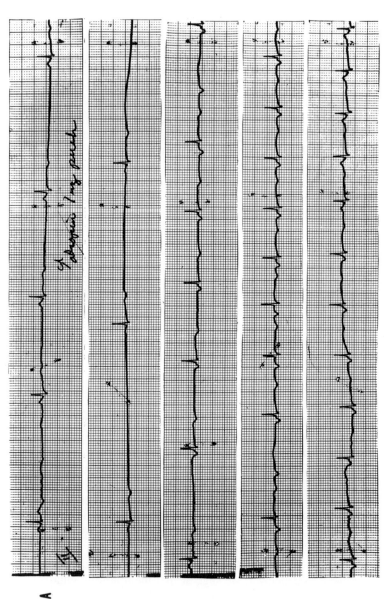

Fig. 18A. A continuous rhythm strip demonstrating extreme sinus bradycardia of 30 beats per minute. Atropine, 1 mgm, was administered (arrow) while the patient was being prepared for a transvenous pacemaker. The rhythm changed transiently to a slow nodal at 44 beats per minute, accelerating to 75 beats per minute, and finally converting spontaneously to sinus rhythm at 88 beats per minute.

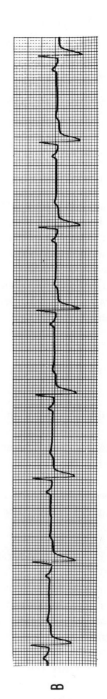

B

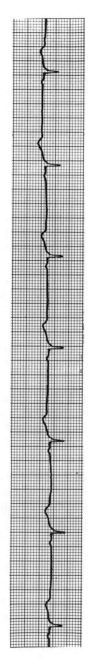

Fig. 18B. Sinus bradycardia associated with inferior wall infarction characteristically presents with heart rates between 40 and 60 beats per minute as shown above. If the ventricular rate cannot be accelerated with atropine sulfate a demand-type pacemaker should be inserted. Heart rates persistently below 50 beats per minute should be paced to 65 beats per minute.

Sinus bradyarrhythmia (unresponsive to atropine)
Heart block (2° or 3°)
Junction rhythm
Bilateral bundle branch block
Inferior infarction with BBB
Anterior infarction with BBB
Changing conducting mechanisms

SINUS BRADYCARDIA

The etiology of sinus bradycardia is not completely understood. The "sick sinus node" is a reflection of ischemic heart disease, acute or chronic. The bradyarrhythmias are seen mainly in inferior or posterior wall infarctions. There appears to be increased vagatonia and increased sensitivity of the sinus node to vagal stimulus. Vagolytic drugs such as atropine offset some vagal action and often reverse sinus bradycardia altogether. Cardiac rates as low as 30 per minute are sometimes seen. Rates below 50 demand immediate attention (Figs. 18A, 18B, and 19).

MANAGEMENT OF THE PATIENT WITH SINUS BRADYCARDIA AND VENTRICULAR RATE BELOW 50

1. Analgesia with morphine sulfate should be avoided unless prescribed in conjection with atropine.
2. Vagal stimulation, e.g., gastric irritation, rectal examination, enemas, etc., should be avoided during the first few days of myocardial infarction.
3. Atropine. A dose of 0.4 mg is prescribed intravenously. It may be repeated every 10 minutes to a maximum of 2.0 mg. The effect of the atropine lasts for 30 to 40 minutes.

If atropine does accelerate the heart rate, and it generally does, an intravenous drip is set up containing 2.0 mg per 500 cc. The speed of the infusion is then set so that the heart rate remains over 60. If not effective, insert the electric pacemaker. We do not advocate the use of isoproterenol at this point. It will accelerate the rate. However, oxygen consumption becomes disproportionately high.

Electric pacemaker. If the intravenous atropine in the dose recommended above fails to accelerate the heart rate, an electric pacemaker should be used. A "demand" type power source is used and the demand rate set to 65. The sinus bradycardia rarely lasts more than a few days.

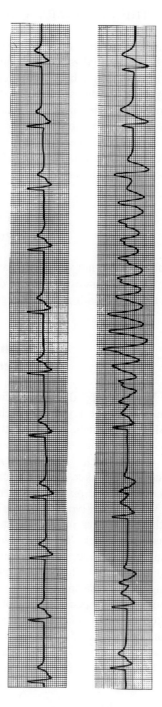

Fig. 19. The effect of untreated bradycardia is demonstrated. Slow ventricular rates from any cause permit the appearance of escape rhythms. In the above continuous rhythm strip, a ventricular rate of 48 beats per minute is associated with a burst of ventricular tachycardia after two ventricular premature beats in the lower strip.

131

The psychological reaction to the thought of having a heart attack, the excitement of being hospitalized and monitored, of being placed on "critical," and in some cases being anointed for the "last rites," should arouse tachycardia in almost everyone. Some have felt that the "normal" pulse under these circumstances should be 70 to 80 at least, and anything less than 70 be considered "coronary brady-arrhythmia." This phrase is introduced here to alert the physician to the idea that serious degrees of bradycardia may be forewarned by the relatively slow rate of 70 when the patient is first seen.

First Degree Heart Block

First degree A-V block does not need special management. Although it may be a forerunner of more advanced degrees of A-V block, the sequence does not occur with sufficient regularity to warrant direct intervention.

Second Degree Heart Block

Second degree heart block (dropped beats) occurs in a variety of forms. The most common are Type I (Wenckebach) and Type II (Moebitz) (Fig. 20). Most physicians feel that the presence of non-conducted sinus beats of the Moebitz type represent impending disaster (bilateral bundle branch block) and represent a clear indication for placing the electric pacemaker. There is some controversy over whether the pacemaker should be placed in patients with second degree heart block of the Wenckebach type. Until this problem is settled, we prefer to place the pacemaker in all patients with dropped beats due to second degree heart block. Transient Wenckebach phenomenon lasting a few minutes or hours is common. Wenckebach episodes lasting for more than 4 to 6 hours generally will persist. We feel this justifies placing the I.V. pacemaker.

In most patients in our series the pacemaker is placed during the first hospital day. Wenckebach phenomenon occurring later in the course (3rd to 4th day) in the absence of any suggestion of extension of the infarction is considered by some to be of less significance as a warning of approaching CHB than that occurring on day 1. We continue to feel that the electric pacemaker wire should be placed at any

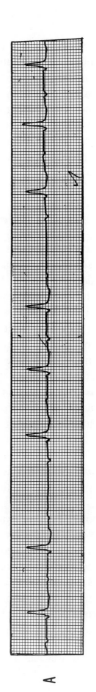

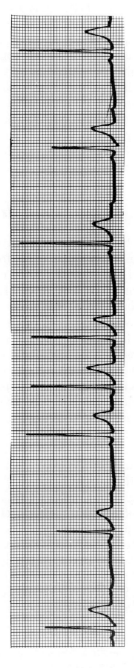

Fig. 20. Second degree heart block is characterized by an intermittent failure of sinus node impulses to reach the ventricles. Wenckebach block (A) is characterized by a progressive delay of impulse transmission through the A-V node, represented by progressive lengthening of the P-R interval, until an impulse fails to traverse the junctional tissue (block), represented by a P wave without a QRS complex. Moebitz block (B) is characterized by an intermittent failure of conduction through junctional tissue, represented by P waves without QRS complexes and normal conduction in the remaining beats. Second degree heart block may suddenly progress to complete heart block. A demand pacemaker should be inserted.

A

B

133

time during the hospital course in the presence of second degree heart block. Under the circumstance of second degree heart block as above, we again emphasize that two decisions are to be made: one, to place the electric pacemaker wire, the other to turn on the electricity. We prefer to place the wire *now*, to remove it if it is not used, rather than try to place it in a crisis situation. We consider this a conservative approach. The same principles hold for *junctional rhythm*. It is unusual to have to actually pace the ventricle for more than 4 days. The longest period we have had to pace has been 11 days.

Complete Heart Block

Complete heart block occurs in 5 to 10 percent of patients with myocardial infarction. Its duration varies from seconds to days and rarely is it permanent. The resulting heart rate depends on the location of the junctional pacemaker (Fig. 21). The higher the pacemaker in the junctional tissue, the faster the rate. Idioventricular rhythm with rates between 30 and 40 result when no viable junctional tissue assumes the function of pacemaker. The earlier one sees patients after the onset of the infarction, the more likely one sees complete heart block. The mortality of complete heart block from several large series before pacemaker therapy was over 50 percent. A 4 to 6 percent incidence of complete heart block documented in patients hospitalized and observed after the first hospital day does not reflect the high mortality of this block on day 1 and in patients who never reach the hospital. *The greatest incidence of heart block in our patients is in those seen in the Emergency Room.* Most frequently, our patients with CHB go from Emergency Room to the catheterizaation lab before going to the Coronary Care Unit.

The diagnosis of complete heart block should be synonymous with the use of a temporary transvenous pacemaker. There is no need for bedside debate about treatment. This does not negate the potential usefulness of drug therapy but supplants it since the surest way to control the ventricular rate is by electrical means. At the first sign of complete heart block a pacemaker should be inserted. If the ventricular rate is below 50 the pacemaker should be turned on and the heart paced at about 65 beats per minute.* This should be continued until

---

* Using the fixed rate pacer. If a "demand" pacemaker is available it should be used and also set "on demand" at about 65.

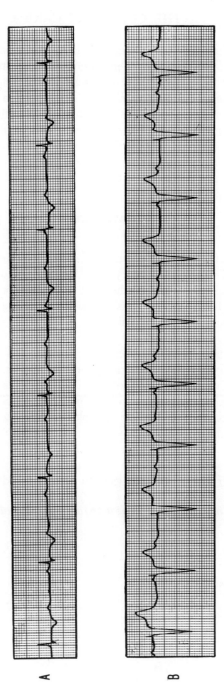

Fig. 21. Complete heart block is shown in rhythm strip A. The atrial rate at 75 beats per minute is regular and independent of the slow ventricular rate at 45 beats per minute. Complete heart block is life-threatening because the rhythm is unstable, the ventricular rate is slow, and escape rhythm with ventricular fibrillation may occur. A pacemaker is inserted and the heart is paced (B) at 62 beats per minute, a rate fast enough to prevent escape rhythm and ventricular fibrillation.

135

a stable supraventricular rhythm is established. As previously stated, complete heart block is a transient phenomenon in acute myocardial infarction. The first indication that the pacemaker is no longer required is the appearance of a sinus rhythm in competition with the fixed note pacemaker. The pacemaker should be turned off periodically and the underlying rhythm observed. When sinus rhythm reappears the pacemaker is turned off or set "on demand" and the rhythm monitored. If sinus rhythm persists for 24 hours the pacemaker may be removed. Once sinus rhythm is established, heart block has not reappeared in our experience.

COMPLETE HEART BLOCK: CURRENT NOTIONS AND EXPERIENCE

The data tabulated below is a summary of our experience with heart block since we began a Coronary Care Unit. Since some transient instances can easily escape recording, the numbers represent the minimum number. These are patients without shock and without heart failure prior to pacing (see Table 1). Keeping in mind our thoughts on mortality rates (Chapter 1, p. 10), which emphasize the necessity for having large numbers of cases, it becomes apparent that much work needs to be done before definitive information on heart block is available. Even though our total series of patients is large, and it represents practically all the patients in the hospital and not only selected patients, the number of examples of any one type of block is still too small for statistical evaluation. The data indicate that complete heart block and "nodal" rhythm carry a very high mortality and in this series the location of the pacemaker (either ventricular or at a higher level) does not seem to make much difference.

TABLE 1. *Pacing in Acute Myocardial Infarction: Total Results*

RHYTHM	TOTAL CASES	TOTAL PACED	AVERAGE HEART RATE	% MORTALITY
CHB				
Ventricular Pacemaker	25	21	37	64
Junctional Pacemaker	18	13	56	50
2° Heart Block	15	11	53	7
Sinus Rhythm	27	18	59	22
Nodal Rhythm	16	9	54	56
Miscellaneous (usually rapidly changing rhythm	14	10	59	64
Totals	115	82	52	43

COMPLETE HEART BLOCK: LOCATION OF PACEMAKER

Table 2 shows the very high mortality rates in complete heart block. On examination of these data it becomes apparent that the location of the infarct is of far more significance in mortality than the location of the pacemaker. Anterior infarction with complete heart block is a large infarction and is associated with almost 100 percent mortality. Inferior infarcts are probably smaller infarcts and are generally associated with lower mortality rates. The high mortality rates in CHB do not seem to be related to the site of the ventricular pacemaker (Tables 2 and 3), as manifested by right bundle branch block or left bundle branch block, as much as they are related to the location of the infarction and its size.

COMPLETE HEART BLOCK: CARDIAC ARREST

The mortality rate of patients with complete heart block who had cardiac arrest was almost 100 percent. (Five of five with junctional pacemakers, nine of nine with ventricular pacemakers). Patients with second and third degree heart block, sinus bradycardia, and nodal rhythm, who had the pacemaker placed in the absence of a cardiac arrest, had an overall mortality of 33 percent. We feel that the high mortality rate in complete heart block is a clear indication for placing the intravenous pacemaker, especially when considering

TABLE 2. *Pacing in Acute Myocardial Infarction: Complete Heart Block*

	JUNCTIONAL PACEMAKER		VENTRICULAR PACEMAKER	
Total Cases		18		25
Dead		9		16
Infarct Location	Anterior	5 – 4 Dead	Anterior	9 – 8 Dead
	Inferior	11 – 3 Dead	Inferior	11 – 6 Dead
	Unknown	2 – 2 Dead	Non-Transmural	2 – 0 Dead
			Unknown	3 – 2 Dead
Conduction Defect	RBBB	6 – 4 Dead	RBBB	9 – 5 Dead
	LBBB	2 – 1 Dead	LBBB	4 – 4 Dead
	None	10 – 4 Dead	IVCD	12 – 7 Dead
Code 99 Prior to Pacing	5 Cases – 5 Dead		9 Cases – 8 Dead	

TABLE 3. *Pacing for Heart Block in Acute Myocardial Infarction: Factors Affecting Mortality*

INFARCT LOCATION	No.	% MORTALITY
Anteroseptal	17	65
Anterior	20	55
Inferior	57	35
Unknown	10	60
Non-Transmural	11	18
CONDUCTION DEFECT	No.	% MORTALITY
RBBB	14	64
RBBB-LAD	11	45
LBBB	14	79
None	76	33

Resuscitation Prior to Pacemaker
28 Cases   Mortality 75%

No Resuscitation Prior to Pacemaker
87 Cases   Mortality 33%

our experience with those patients who needed cardiac resuscitation before the pacemaker was placed.

BUNDLE BRANCH BLOCK (BBB)

Bundle branch block occurs in approximately 10 percent of collected series (A.H.A. reports). However, Stock reports an incidence of almost 25 percent. BBB is not often related to A-V block although it is frequently classified with A-V block.

Of considerable interest is the variety of BBB-RBBB QV_1 which has been clearly identified with CHB and causes a high mortality. (See following section.) The high mortality in BBB is probably due to the fact that BBB represents an extensive infarction and/or a strategically placed infarct. If the lesion is a large infarction, the mortality rate will be high. If it is strategically located in such a way as to

TABLE 4. *Therapy in Sinus Bradycardia and Heart Block*

ELECTRIC PACEMAKER	ELECTRIC PACEMAKER OR DRUG THERAPY
Bilateral BBB	A-V Block
CHB	Sinus Bradycardia
BBB	Nodal Rhythm
2°HB (Moebitz)	2°HB (Wenckebach)

induce bilateral BBB, death may ensue from CHB and asystole. The feeling is growing among those who supervise CCU's, that BBB is a serious sign. It may be the only warning of impending complete heart block in patients with anterior infarction, or may be the indicator of bilateral bundle branch block in patients with inferior infarction (RBBBQV₁).

BILATERAL BUNDLE BRANCH BLOCK

The electrocardiogram showing acute RBBB in the V leads, Q waves in V_1–V_3, and left axis deviation carries a high mortality rate (Fig. 22). This ECG is interpreted as indicating involvement of the right bundle and the anterior superior division of the left bundle. We were able to find nine instances of this in our patients after learning of this phenomenon through Dr. Richard Stock. Our nine patients died in asystole without prior second or third degree heart block. Since then we have placed the I.V. pacemaker in such patients as soon as we recognized the ECG pattern, and we have had two survivors.

DRUG THERAPY OF COMPLETE HEART BLOCK

There are advocates of drug therapy in complete heart block, but drugs are considered by most to represent interim therapy until the patient has a pacemaker inserted (Table 4).

Isoproterenol (Isuprel). This is undoubtedly the drug of choice for accelerating heart rates in complete heart block. For short-term use it is extremely effective and also provides a positive inotropic force. The beta adrenergic property of isoproterenol is hazardous for prolonged therapy because of the metabolic demands it imposes on mitochondria. The oxygen debt cannot be paid by a compromised pump. The vasodilatation which accompanies isoproterenol therapy lowers blood pressure which is a critical factor in coronary perfusion. The usual dose of the drug is 2 mg (1 ampule) in 500 cc of dextrose solution with titration of the dose until a therapeutic effect is noted. It may be administered during the brief time it takes to transport the patient to an area where the pacemaker is inserted. *Isoproterenol must be discontinued before pacing is begun.* The concomitant use of the drug and electric cardiac pacing results in severe tachyarrhythmias which may prove resistant to all forms of therapy.

Corticosteroids. The rationale for steroid therapy is based on its anti-inflammatory properties. Lev has conclusively demonstrated that

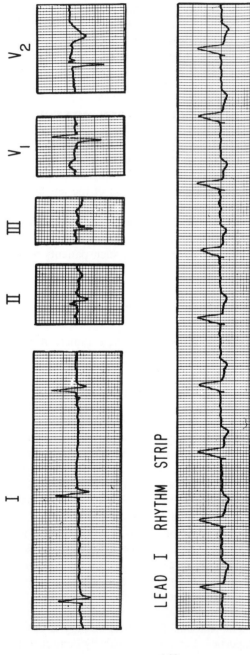

LEAD I RHYTHM STRIP

Fig. 22. A type of bilateral bundle branch block commonly associated with bradycardia, complete heart block, and asystole is shown. This syndrome is characterized by left axis deviation, right bundle branch block, and Q waves in leads V_1 and V_2. A demand pacemaker should always be inserted in such situations, since asystole and heart block frequently ensue. Note in Lead I above the extreme bradycardia at 42 beats per minute and the rhythm strip showing pacemaker rhythm at 64 beats per minute.

the conduction pathways are not destroyed in acute heart block. The cause of heart block in AMI is thought to be local inflammation in the region of the A-V node or His bundle. The rewarding results of steroid administration in such diverse situations as cerebral edema and sarcoidosis of the heart has prompted their use in heart block with, at times, seemingly good results. Steroids have also an accelerator effect on conduction tissue. The effect of steroids on serum potassium concentration may be important. Solu Medrol or its equivalent is given in a dose of 4 cc every 6 hours intravenously. If steroids reverse heart block, they do so within 2 hours. They may be prescribed after the pacemaker wire is inserted but their continued use is unjustified. The authors have no confidence in steroids for heart block and permit their use only as long as it takes to insert the electric pacemaker.

ECTOPIC RHYTHMS IN THE PRESENCE OF HEART BLOCK

Escape rhythms may appear when the heart rate is slow. Ventricular tachycardia is the most fearsome result because of its usual progression to ventricular fibrillation. Other ectopic rhythms may appear such as premature ventricular contraction.

Antiarrhythmic drugs are contraindicated for ectopic arrhythmias in the presence of heart block or other bradyarrhythmias.

Antiarrhythmic drugs depress impulse formation in the A-V node as well as conduction through junctional tissue and the ventricles. The only pacemaker the patient has may be suppressed with antiarrhythmic drugs. The treatment of ectopic rhythms in the face of bradycardia is aimed to accelerate the ventricular rate above that "critical" rate which will impede ectopic impulse formation. If after acceleration of the ventricular rate, PVC's continue to appear, xylocaine may be prescribed as a 50 mg bolus. Quinidine-like drugs should be avoided in heart block or any bradyarrhythmia. If ventricular tachycardia complicates heart block the arrhythmia should be cardioverted and the ventricular rate again controlled by electric pacing.

ATRIAL FIBRILLATION IN CHB

An unusual rhythm, atrial fibrillation and CHB, has occasionally been recorded. Here the treatment is placing of the electric pacemaker as in any heart block and ventricular pacing if the ventricular rate drops below 50. Digitalis toxicity should always be considered when this arrhythmia is seen.

Summary

A-V block is common in acute myocardial infarction Electric pacing is the management of choice in third degree heart block and in second degree heart block. For first degree heart block no special therapy is needed. Drug therapy followed by pacing is necessary in cases of marked sinus bradycardia. Mortality rates are very high in patients with CHB. Present knowledge in BBB is grossly inadequate; however, electric pacing in some of these patients may be indicated to anticipate A-V dissociation due to bilateral BBB. Much work must be done and much data need to be accumulated before definition of treatment of heart block can be stated. In the meantime, the authors feel that electric pacing using a demand pacemaker is "conservative" treatment and is safe.

References

Adgey, J., Geddes, J. S., Mulholland, H. C., Keegan, P. A. J., and Pantridge, J. F. Incidence, significance, and management of early bradyarrhythmia complicating acute myocardial infarction. Lancet, 2:1097, 1968.

——— Nelson, P. G., Scott, M. E., Geddes, J. S., Allen, J. D., Zaidi, S. A., and Pantridge, J. F. Management of ventricular fibrillation outside hospital. Lancet, 1:1169, 1969.

Ayres, S. M., and Grace, W. J. Inappropriate ventilation and hypoxemia as causes of cardiac arrhythmia. Amer. J. Med., 46:495, 1969.

Bacaner, M. B. Quantitative comparison of Bretylium with other antifibrillatory drugs. Amer. J. Cardiol., 21:504, 1968.

——— Treatment of ventricular fibrillation and other acute arrythmias with Bretylium Tosylate. Amer. J. Cardiol., 21:530, 1968.

Barold, S. S., and Center, S. Electrocardiographic diagnosis of perforation of the heart by pacing catheter electrode. Amer. J. Cardiol., 24:274, 1969.

Beck, C. S., Pritchard, W. H., and Feil, H. S. Ventricular fibrillation of long duration abolished by electric shock. J.A.M.A., 135:985, 1947.

Beregovich, J., Fenig, S., Lasser, J., and Allen, D. Management of myocardial infarction complicated by advanced atrioventricular block. Amer. J. Cardiol., 23:54, 1969.

Bilitch, M., Cosby, R. C., and Cafferky, E. A. Ventricular fibrillation and competitive pacing. New Eng. J. Med., 276:598, 1967.

Brown, K. W. G., MacMillan, R. L., Forbath, N., Mel'Grano, F., and Scott, J. W. Coronary unit—an intensive care center for acute myocardial infarction. Lancet, 2:349, 1963.

Bruce, R. A., Blackmon, J. R., Cobb, L. A., and Dodge, H. T. Treatment of asystole or heart block during acute myocardial infarction with electrode catheter pacemaking. Amer. Heart J., 69:460, 1965.

Campion, B. C., Harrison, C. E., Jr., Giuliani, E. R., Schattenberg, T. T., Ellis, F. H., Jr. Ventricular septal defect after myocardial infarction. Ann. Int. Med., 70:251, 1969.

Castellanos, A. C., Lemberg, L., Scheib, R. J., Budkin, A. Cardioversion of A-V nodal tachycardia. Amer. J. Cardiol., 18:884, 1966.

———— Lemberg, L., and Fanseca, E. J. Ventricular arrhythmias after D.C. countershock. Amer. Heart J., 70:583, 1965.

Chatterjee, K., Harris, A., and Leatham, A. The risk of pacing after infarction, and current recommendations. Lancet, 2:1061, 1969.

Conrad, J. K., Mowry, F. M., and Juan, L. L. Transvenous pacing in two patients with repetitive ventricular arrhythmia. Arch. Int. Med., 122:507, 1968.

Day, H. W., and Averill, K. Recorded arrhythmias in an acute coronary care area. Dis. Chest, 49:113, 1966.

Donoso, E., Cohn, L. J., and Freidberg, C. K. Ventricular arrhythmias after precordial electric shock. Amer. Heart J., 73:595, 1967.

Fluck, D. C., Olsen, B., Pentecost, B. L., Thomas, M., Filmore, S. J., Shillingford, J. P., and Mounsey, I. P. D. Natural history and clinical significance of arrhythmia after acute myocardial infarction. Brit. Heart J., 29:170, 1967.

Frieden, J., Rosenblum, R., Enselberg, C. D., and Rosenberg, A. Propranolol treatment of chronic intractable supraventricular arrhythmias. Amer. J. Cardiol., 22:711, 1968.

Goetz, R. H., Goldstein, J. V., Frater, R. W. M., and Berkovits, B. Demand pacing in intermittent heart block. J.A.M.A., 205:657, 1968.

Gregory, J. J., and Grace, W. J. The management of sinus bradycardia, nodal rhythm and heart block for the prevention of cardiac arrest in acute myocardial infarction. Prog. Cardiovasc. Dis., 10:505, 1968.

Hahn, J., DeTragila, J., Millet, D., and Moe, G. The incidence of ectopic beats as a function of the basic rate in the ventricle. Amer. Heart J., 72:632, 1966.

———— Malozzi, A. M., and Lyons, C. Ventricular vulnerability to paired-pulse stimulation during acute coronary occlusion. Amer. Heart J., 73:79, 1967.

Jewitt, D. E., Balcon, R., Raftery, E. B., and Oram, S. Incidence and management of supraventricular arrhythmias after acute myocardial infarction. Lancet, 2:734, 1968.

Julian, D. G., Valentine, P. A., and Miller, G. G. Disturbances of rate, rhythm and conduction in acute myocardial infarction. Amer. J. Med., 37:915, 1964.

Kahler, R. L., Burrow, G. N., and Felig, P. Diazepam induced amnesia for cardioversion. J.A.M.A., 200:189, 1967.

Katz, L., and Pick, A. Clinical Electrocardiography. Philadelphia, Lea & Febiger, 1956.

Killip, T., and Gault, J. H. Mode of onset of atrial fibrillation in man. Amer. Heart J., 29:575, 1965.

Kimball, J. T., and Killip, T. Aggressive treatment of arrhythmias in acute myocardial infarction. Prog. Cardiovasc. Dis., 10:483, 1968.

Kleiger, R., and Lown, B. Cardioversion and digitalis. Circulation, 33:878, 1966.

Konttinen, A., Hupli, V., Lauhija, A., and Gottfried, H. Elevated serum enzyme activity after direct-current countershock. New Eng. J. Med., 281:231, 1969.

Kouwenhoven, W. B., and Kay, J. H. A simple electrical apparatus for the treatment of ventricular fibrillation. Surgery, 30:781, 1951.

Langendorf, R., Pick, A., and Winternitz, M. Mechanisms of intermittment ventricular bigeminy. Appearance of ectopic beats dependent upon length of ventricular cycle, the rule of bigeminy. Circulation, 11:422, 1955.

Lemberg, L., Castellanos, A., and Berkovits, B. Pacemaking on demand in A-V block. J.A.M.A., 191:106, 1965.

Lewis, A. J., Burchell, H. B., and Titus, J. L. Clinical and pathologic features of post infarction cardiac rupture. Amer. J. Cardiol., 23:43, 1969.

Lewis, T. Diseases of the Heart, 3rd ed. London, MacMillan Company, 1943, p.98.

Lister, J. W., Damato, A. N., Kosowsky, B. D., Lau, S. H., and Stein, E. The hemodynamic effect of slowing the heart rate by paired or coupled stimulation of the atria. Amer. Heart J., 73:362, 1967.

Lown B., Amarasingham, R., and Neumann, J. A. A new method for terminating cardiac arrhythmias. Use of synchronized capacitor discharge. J.A.M.A., 182:548, 1962.

—— Kleiger, R., and Wolff, G. The technique of cardioversion. Amer. Heart J., 67:282, 1964.

—— and Levine, S. A. The carotid sinus: Clinical value of its stimulation. Circulation, 23:766, 1961.

—— Neumann, J., Amarasingham, R., and Berkovits, B. V. Comparison of alternating current with direct electroshock across the closed chest. Amer. J. Cardiol., 10:233, 1962.

—— and Vassaux, C. Lidocaine in acute myocardinal infarction. Amer. Heart J., 76:586, 1968.

Marriott, J. L. Simulation of ectopic ventricular rhythms by aberrant conduction. J.A.M.A., 196:787, 1966.

Meltzer, L. E., and Kitchell, J. B. Arrhythmias and acute myocardial infarction. Prog. Cardiovasc. Dis., 9:50, 1966.

Mounsey, P. Intensive coronary care, Arrhythmias after acute myocardial infarction. Amer. J. Cardiol., 20:475, 1967.

Pamfret, D., Polansky, B. J., and Huvos, A. Dangerous complication of temporary floating pacing electrodes. New Eng. J. Med., 280:651, 1969.

Paulk, E. A., and Hurst, J. W. Complete heart block in acute myocardial infarction. Amer. J. Cardiol., 17:695, 1966.

Rossi, M., and Lown, B. The use of quinidine in cardioversion. Amer. J. Cardiol., 19:234, 1966.

Shillingford, J., and Thomas, M. Treatment of bradycardia and hypotension syndrome in patients with acute myocardial infarction. Amer. Heart J., 75:843, 1968.

Smirk, F. H., and Palmer, D. G. A myocardial syndrome. With particular reference to the occurrence of sudden death and premature systoles interrupting antecedent T waves. Amer. J. Cardiol., 6:620, 1960.

Spann, J. F., Moellering, R. C., Jr., Haber, E., and Wheeler, E. Arrhythmias in acute myocardial infarction. New Eng. J. Med., 271:427, 1964.

Stock, E. Arrhythmias after myocardial infarction. Amer. Heart J., 75:435, 1968.

—— Goble, A., and Sloman, G. Assessment of arrhythmias in myocardial infarction. Brit. Med. J., 2:719, 1967.

—— and Macken, D. L. Observations on heart block during continuous electrocardiographic monitoring in myocardial infarction. Circulation, 38:993, 1969.

Stock, J. P. P. Beta adrenergic blocking drugs in the clinical management of cardiac arrhythmia. Amer. J. Cardiol., 18:444, 1966.

Stock, R. J., and Macken, D. L. Observations on heart block during continuous electrocardiographic monitoring in myocardial infarction. Circulation, 37:993, 1968.

Thomas, M., and Woodgate, D. Effect of atropine on bradycardia and hypotension in acute myocardial infarction. Brit. Heart J., 28:409, 1966.

Tsagaris, T. J., Bustamante, R. A., and Friesendorf, R. A. Unusual complication of transvenous electrical pacing of the heart. Dis. Chest, 53:110, 1968.

Vassaux, C., and Lown, B. Cardioversion of supraventricular tachycardias. Circulation, 39:791, 1969.

——— and Lown, B. Myocardial infarction and the vulnerable period for ventricular tachycardia. Clin. Res., 15:255, 1967.

Warbase, J. R., Wesley, J. E., Connolly, V., and Galluzzi, N. J. Lactic dehydrogenase isoenzymes after electroshock treatment of cardiac arrhythmias. Amer. J. Cardiol., 21:496, 1968.

Zoll, P. M., Linethal, A. J., Gibson, W., Paul, M. H., and Norman, L. R. Termination of ventricular fibrillation in man by externally applied electric counter shock. New Eng. J. Med., 254:727, 1956.

6

Congestive Heart Failure

Congestive heart failure, one of the most serious complications of acute myocardial infarction, causes 20 percent of the fatalities. It is as serious a complication as shock and accordingly must be treated vigorously. The incidence of congestive heart failure in acute myocardial infarction varies depending on the criteria for the diagnosis of heart failure. The incidence ranges from 5 to 10 percent when pulmonary edema alone is considered to 80 to 90 percent when rales at the lung bases are included. Heart failure may be a feature of other complications, such as arrhythmias and shock. Isolated congestive heart failure is unusual in acute myocardial infarction.

Varieties of Congestive
Heart Failure

There are two clinical syndromes classified under congestive heart failure: 1) acute pulmonary edema, and 2) classic congestive heart failure.*

1) Acute pulmonary edema is a clinical entity that represents the result of extreme left ventricular failure. The typical patient is alarmingly short of breath. A prominent cough is present. Sputum production varies from very little to profuse watery blood-stained "froth." The patient is acutely ill, cyanotic, diaphoretic, and generally agitated. Tachycardia, distended neck veins and a ventricular diastolic gallop (S_3 gallop) are prominent. Hepatomegaly and peripheral edema may be present. Diffuse crepitant rales are present in the lung fields. Pulmonary edema may be the initial presenting feature of acute myocardial infarction or may appear hours to days later during the course of the illness. It is unusual for pulmonary edema to be the initial presenting feature of a patient's first myocardial infarction unless complicated by diabetes or hypertension.

2) Congestive heart failure (classic) is a clinical entity due to variable but lesser degrees of left ventricular failure Compared with acute pulmonary edema, congestive heart failure presents a more insidious onset and manifests milder symptoms of dyspnea. Orthopnea is unusual. While tachycardia and gallop rhythm are usually observed, rales in the lung fields are less diffuse and sometimes limited only to the bases. Hepatomegaly and edema are variable with

* Pump failure is a term coined in the past decade. The term is loosely associated with both congestive heart failure and shock. Shock and congestive heart failure are probably variants and extremes of pump failure. "Power failure" is another term frequently used. As defined, power failure represents that peculiar syndrome encountered after a heart has been defibrillated when electrical activity is present but no mechanical activity can be detected. We have no explanation for this phenomenon. Power failure is sometimes encountered with ruptured ventricle, more often it is seen with an intact ventricle after resuscitative efforts.

There appears to be no value in considering pump failure as a separate clinical entity. Too few patients have been studied thoroughly to warrant naming a new syndrome. The addition of new terminology adds little to our understanding of the mechanism of heart failure. We prefer to consider heart failure in the traditional sense until such time as new information and physiologic data warrant the distinction of "power" and "pump" failure from congestive heart failure.

their extent proportional to the duration of congestive heart failure. Classic congestive heart failure may be the initial presenting feature of acute myocardial infarction but more commonly it appears later in the course of illness.

Hemodynamics of Heart Failure in Acute Myocardial Infarction

All patients with acute myocardial infarction have heart failure in the sense that the cardiac output is reduced because of a reduced capacity to eject blood from the left ventricle because of the infarcted muscle. Left ventricular end-diastolic pressure is elevated and is reflected by pulmonary vascular congestion. This produces physiologic shunting of blood with a lowered arterial oxygen tension. Left ventricular failure may cause right ventricular failure which leads to peripheral edema. Left ventricular failure may also cause pulmonary edema leading to right ventricular failure. Acute myocardial infarction is rarely associated with isolated right ventricular failure. While the cardiac output is somewhat lowered in acute myocardial infarction, it is not always necessary or wise to treat all cases with digitalis.

Differential Diagnosis

SERUM ENZYMES IN ACUTE PULMONARY EDEMA

The syndrome of congestive heart failure is simple to diagnose but its relationship to myocardial infarction is not always clear. Patients who suffer myocardial infarction do not all develop congestive heart failure. More importantly, all patients who experience acute pulmonary edema have not suffered an acute myocardial infarction. Differentiation may be based on the level of the serum enzymes.

Routine measurements of serum enzymes include the serum glutamic oxalacetic acid (SGOT), the serum lactic dehydrogenase (LDH) and the serum creatine pyruvic kinase (CPK). Every laboratory should include the CPK for the proper diagnosis of myocardial infarction. The isozymes of LDH have not consistently been shown to distinguish hepatic, pulmonary, and cardiac damage. While SGOT and

LDH are frequently elevated in pulmonary edema or congestive heart failure due to passive congestion of the liver, the serum CPK is elevated only when cardiac or skeletal muscle or brain tissue is damaged. Thus elevated levels of CPK in pulmonary edema suggest the presence of acute myocardial infarction (in the absence of obvious trauma or CNS disease).

In evaluating our patients with pulmonary edema we accept a rise in the serum CPK level to twice the normal level as evidence of myocardial injury. For example, the normal range of serum CPK by our autoanalyzer technique is 15 to 80 units. A serum CPK of from 90 to 140 units is equivocal evidence of myocardial injury in the absence of skeletal muscle injury. Levels of greater than 150 units are definite evidence of myocardial injury. Similarly, serum levels of SGOT and LDH must be twice normal to be considered unequivocal evidence of infarction. In our experience the serum enzymes are elevated from 2 to 5 times normal in acute myocardial infarction. Caution must be exercised when evaluating a patient who has been cardioverted or defibrillated as these procedures themselves produce a massive rise in the serum enzymes without infarction.

Treatment of Pulmonary Edema

The treatment of pulmonary edema requires prompt, diligent, and continuous professional care. The primary defect is left ventricular failure and treatment is directed toward alleviating the results of this failure until the myocardium compensates. Specific therapeutic procedures include positive pressure oxygen, morphine sulfate, rotating tourniquets, and phlebotomy.

MORPHINE SULFATE

Morphine sulfate continues to be the anchor in the chain of prescriptions for pulmonary edema. The exact mechanism of action is not understood. For the average sized man from 10-15 mg are prescribed initially, subcutaneously or intramuscularly. There is rarely a need to prescribe morphine sulfate intravenously. When because of profound hypotension morphine must be given I.V., only one-third dose should be administered by vein and the remaining two-thirds given I.M. If after 20 to 30 minutes the patient continues to be tachypneic and agitated, the dose of morphine may be repeated. More than 60 mg should never be given in a one-hour period!

DIURETICS-TOURNIQUETS-PHLEBOTOMY

Diuretics, phlebotomy and rotating tourniquets may be grouped together because the net result is the same, the removal of fluid from the right side of the circulation. The introduction of furosemide and ethacrynic acid in the past few years has almost removed phlebotomy from the armamentarium. These potent diuretic drugs produce an "autophlebotomy." Their intravenous administration produces a prompt diuresis in 15 minutes and the excretion of as much as 2 liters of urine in the first hour. Furosemide and ethacrynic acid offer no more than mercurial diuretics after an 8-hour period but their prompt action makes them more suitable in the treatment of pulmonary edema. Both furosemide and ethacrynic acid are administered intravenously. They may be prescribed orally but in pulmonary edema prompt action is desired and for this reason they are prescribed intravenously. The initial dose of furosemide is 40 mg which may be repeated every half-hour. Massive doses have been prescribed, as much as 1000 mg orally per day, with no deleterious effect. The safety of more than 200 mg intravenously has not been established. The dose of ethacrynic acid is 50 mg to start and is repeated in 15 minutes if no effect is noted. Single doses of more than 100 mg intravenously may produce profound changes in fluid and electrolyte balance and should be reserved for extreme emergencies. Venous phlebotomy is rarely if ever necessary in acute pulmonary edema.

Rotating tourniquets remove blood from the circulation by trapping it in the extremities. The technique of rotating tourniquets is time-consuming but may be effective. Rubber tubing is snugly applied to the proximal end of three extremities. Every 15 minutes all the tourniquets are loosened and re-applied to three other extremities, thus rotating a free extremity. It is imperative to loosen all the tourniquets, otherwise each extremity will have a tourniquet applied to it for 45 continuous minutes. A sphygmomanometer cuff is preferred to rubber straps. The pressure should be set between the systolic and diastolic blood pressure levels. Machines are now available which automatically "rotate" the tourniquets once the cuffs are applied and the time interval and pressure are prescribed. Rotating tourniquets are used concurrently in desperate situations. This therapy is used less often now that potent and effective diuretic drugs are available.

Positive pressure oxygen therapy should be immediately instituted in all cases of pulmonary edema. If the patient is conscious and cooperative, oxygen under pressure may be delivered by a snugly fitting face mask. If the patient is hypotensive, unconscious or severely agitated, intubation with a cuffed endotracheal tube should be instituted followed by positive pressure oxygen therapy. Positive pressure is applied by adding a retard cap to any system of oxygen administration. A face mask and bag or a volume-cycled respirator can easily be adapted with a retard cap. The cap is set to the opening of the largest aperture. Every 10 to 15 minutes the aperture size is diminished. This increases peripheral airway resistance and raises intra-alveolar pressure above pulmonary capillary pressure, thus forcing fluid out of the alveolar space and back into the pulmonary circulation. The intra-alveolar oxygen concentration is raised and subsequently Po_2 is raised. In this manner, pulmonary edema can be controlled in about 1 hour. Rapidly decreasing the aperture size of the retard cap may be hazardous. This is manifested by continued agitation of the patient and an increase in tachypnea. If this is observed the next larger aperture is chosen and maintained.

If positive pressure oxygen produced by a retard cap is not sufficient to elevate oxygen tension and control pulmonary edema then a volume-cycled respirator should be used. The volume-cycled respirator (as outlined in other sections) pays several dividends in pulmonary edema. It augments the decrease in venous return to the heart, decreases the work of breathing, and delivers an adequate tidal volume under pressure. In order to institute positive pressure oxygen with a volume-cycled respirator, the patient must be intubated with a cuffed endotracheal tube. This is well tolerated by most patients and remains inserted until the pulmonary edema is corrected. We never perform tracheostomy to deliver positive pressure oxygen in the presence of acute pulmonary edema.

DIGITALIS

Digitalis plays a minor role in the treatment of acute pulmonary edema. Pulmonary edema can usually be controlled before digitalis has time to exert its inotropic effect. If it cannot be controlled within 1 hour after the institution of the preceding regimen, then digitalis should be considered. The rapidly acting drugs, ouabain or cedilanid, are the preparations of choice. The dose of ouabain is 0.1 mg administered slowly intravenously every 15 minutes until a therapeutic effect is noted either by a reduction in cardiac rate, diminution of rales or a lessening of tachypnea. Do not exceed 0.4 mg. The digitalizing dose of cedilanid and digoxin is also reduced in the presence of acute myocardial infarction.

Digitalis should never be administered as a bolus injection. There is ample evidence that the irritability of the myocardium to digitalis is more pronounced in the infarcted heart. Arrhythmia may result from small doses of digitalis in the infarcted heart as compared to the normal.

Treatment of Classic Congestive Heart Failure

Patients with acute myocardial infarction all show some element of left ventricular dysfunction. An S_3 gallop and rales at the lung bases can be heard in most patients with AMI during the first few days of their illness. To treat aggressively all signs and symptoms of left ventricular dysfunction in AMI would be a disservice to the majority of patients. While the ultimate treatment of heart failure has not changed since Withering's classic description of Foxglove, not every sign of congestive failure in acute myocardial infarction requires the prescription of digitalis. Indeed, digitalis may be hazardous to some patients. The following is a tabulation of signs of congestive heart failure which may be treated without digitalis.

1. *Gallop rhythm:* During the first few days of myocardial infarct, an S_3 (ventricular diastolic gallop) can be heard in almost two-thirds of all patients. In some it may persist for many weeks. In most it persists for only a few days and may reappear intermittently during ambulation. An S_4 (atrial diastolic gallop) is likewise heard during the early days of infarction in practically all cases. Of itself a gallop sound is not an indication for digitalis. The S_3 gallop represents ventricular dysfunction and loss of compliance or increased end diastolic pressure in the left ventricle. Only in conjunction with other signs of congestive failure do gallop sounds signify a need for digitalis therapy.

2. *Rales:* Crepitant rales are heard at the posterior bases of the

lung fields in 75 percent of patients with myocardial infarct. Rales are evanescent and disappear completely by the end of the first hospital week. They frequently clear with deep breathing or coughing. Digitalis should be considered when rales are accompanied by dyspnea.

3. *Tachycardia:* As mentioned in another chapter (Arrhythmia), sinus tachycardia is of itself not an indication for digitalis. Most patients have tachycardia in the first few days of hospitalization. Persistent tachycardia with gallop sounds should alert the physician to overt failure and the need for digitalis. Treatment of sinus tachycardia with digitalis in the absence of congestive failure is unnecessary and may be hazardous.

4. *Edema*: This is not seen in the course of acute myocardial infarction unless complicated by long-standing congestive failure. Peripheral edema may be treated with diuretics alone. Mercuhydrin has been the mainstay of diuretic therapy. Two cc (intramuscularly) prescribed every second or third day will control mild to moderate edema. Ethacrynic acid is also effective and may be prescribed by mouth or intravenously, 50 mg twice per day. Total sodium output and free water clearance of ethacrynic acid and mercuhydrin are about the same after 8 hours. Ethacrynic acid offers some advantage in that the onset of action is 15 minutes by the intravenous route and its peak action is reached in 1 hour. Furosemide (Lasix), another potent diuretic, is likewise effective. It may be administered by mouth or intravenously in a dose of 40 to 80 mg once or twice a day.

Congestive failure may be adequately treated with bed rest, oxygen, and diuretics. The judicious use of diuretics may circumvent the need for digitalis or at least postpone its administration to a time when the infarcted heart is less irritable.

DIGITALIS THERAPY IN ACUTE MYOCARDIAL INFARCTION

There are no hard and fast rules for the prescription of digitalis. We have tended to postpone its use until after the first week of illness in acute myocardial infarction. Digitalis is prescribed earlier under the following circumstances.

1. *Dyspnea or tachypnea.* Persistent dyspnea or tachypnea signifies hypoxemia. In conjunction with other signs of congestive heart failure, dyspnea which fails to respond to oxygen therapy should be treated with digitalis.

2. *Atrial fibrillation with a rapid ventricular rate.* When atrial fibrillation is unresponsive to electrical cardioversion (see Arrhythmia), or when cardioversion is contraindicated, ventricular rates above 120/minute should be controlled by digitalis. It is clear that rates above 120/minute hamper ventricular filling and are associated with diminishing cardiac output and, for this reason, the ventricular rate should be controlled. A rate between 90-110/minute is satisfactory. It is not necessary to prescribe large doses of digitalis just to decrease heart rate to 70 beats/minute.

3. *Persistent signs of congestive heart failure which fail to respond to oxygen, bedrest, and diuretics.* There are many methods of prescribing digitalis. Most are based on the concept of a loading dose followed by a maintenance dose. In AMI the loading dose must be reduced to one-half of the usual loading dose. In experimental myocardial infarction in dogs, the toxic dose of digitalis is reduced to 20-30 percent. The toxic dose of digitalis directly injected into the coronary artery is one-twentieth of the toxic dose administered by peripheral vein. The infarcted myocardium is more susceptible to the toxic properties of digitalis (Lown). The dose of digitalis for congestive heart failure in acute myocardial infarction is accordingly reduced. The drug is prescribed in small increments and administered slowly. A bolus injection of any digitalis preparation is contraindicated. It is conceivable that a bolus may arrive at a coronary artery poorly diluted and become a fatal dose to an infarcted heart. There probably is no advantage of one digitalis preparation over another except that theoretically the preparation with a prompt action and rapid excretion is preferable in the event of overdosage. For this reason ouabain has gained wide popularity. Peak action develops within 20 minutes and wanes in 4 hours. Ouabain is prescribed intravenously in doses of 0.1 mg to a total of from 0.3 to 0.5 mg in 1 hour. The time interval between doses depends on the gravity of the situation. It may be as frequent as every 15 minutes or as long as every 4 hours. Each individual dose should be diluted and delivered slowly over a period of 10 minutes. After the last dose of ouabain, digitalization with a modified loading dose of digoxin is begun.

In less critical situations digoxin is a suitable digitalis preparation. The loading dose by mouth is approximately one-half the usual dose or 1.0 mg given over a 2-day period in divided doses. Maintenance therapy is also half the usual dose or 0.125 mg per day. Azotemia and diminished urine output call for a decrease in the above doses of digitalis. Jelliffe has carefully defined the dose of digitalis in the azotemic patient.

Serum electrolytes must be kept at normal levels. Specific attention is paid to the serum potassium. Potassium supplements are given to digitalized patients who receive potent diuretics regardless of the serum potassium levels. Potassium must be prescribed as the chloride salt for proper absorption, retention, and utilization by the intracellular compartment. Elixir of KCl, 15 mEq, 3 times a day orally, is prescribed. If the patient is taking nothing by mouth, KCl, 40 mEq a day, is administered I.V., but never greater than 10 mEq in 1-hour intervals.

PERITONEAL DIALYSIS AND PULMONARY EDEMA

Peritoneal dialysis has proved to be a very useful therapeutic tool in the treatment of acute and chronic renal disease. It is especially useful for the over-hydrated state. A prompt and copious diuresis may be produced by employing hypertonic solutions. Peritoneal dialysis has not received the attention it deserves in the treatment of pulmonary edema. It is a useful adjunct for the occasional patient who fails to respond with a diuresis from drugs because of severely diminished cardiac output and poor renal blood flow. Peritoneal dialysis with hypertonic infusions has been employed five times at St. Vincent's Hospital after failure of the usual therapy for pulmonary edema. In all cases diuresis was achieved. Survival rate did not improve but it is felt that in the future this form of treatment should not be delayed until all hope fails.

References

Cairns, K. B., Porter, G. A., Klasten, F. E., Bristow, J. D., and Griswold, H. E. Clinical and hemodynamic results of peritoneal dialysis for severe cardiac failure. Amer. Heart J., 76:227, 1968.

Gregory, J. J., and Grace, W. J. Resuscitation of the severely ill patient with acute myocardial infarction. Amer. J. Cardiol., 20:836,1967.

Hood, W. B., Jr., Letac, B., Roberge, G., and Lown, B. Direct digitalization of the myocardium: Hemodynamic effects. Amer. J. Cardiol., 22:667, 1968.

Jelliffe, R. W. An improved method of digoxin therapy. Ann. Intern. Med., 69:703, 1968.

Laragh, J. H. Ethacrynic acid and furosemide. Amer. Heart J., 75:564, 1968.

Malach, M. Digitalis for congestive heart failure with heart block in acute myocardial infarction. Amer. Heart J., 76:18, 1968.

Morris, J. J., Taft, C. V., Whalen, R. E., and McIntosh, M. D. Digitalis and experimental myocardial infarction. Amer. Heart J., 77:342, 1969.

Roberge, G., Hood, W. B., and Lown, B. Digitalization of the myocardium in the intact animal by direct coronary artery drug administration. I. Methodologic and pharmacologic considerations. Amer. J. Cardiol., 21:213, 1968.

Sampson, J. J., and Hutchinson, J. C. Heart failure in myocardial infarction. Prog. Cardiovasc. Dis., 10:1, 1968.

Selzer, A. The use of digitalis in acute myocardial infarction. Prog. Cardiovasc. Dis., 10:518, 1968.

Siegel, W., and Gifford, R. W., Jr. Efficacy of ethacrynic acid in patients with refractory congestive heart failure resistant to meralluride. Amer. J. Cardiol., 22:260, 1968.

Vasko. J. S., Henney, P. R., Oldham, N. L., Brawley, R. K., and Morrow, A. G. Mechanisms of action of morphine in the treatment of experimental pulmonary edema. Amer. J. Cardiol., 18:876, 1968.

7

Hypotension and Shock in Acute Myocardial Infarction

Any treatment aimed at the management of acute myocardial infarction in the Coronary Care Unit must concern itself with the problem of shock. Although many patients in the shock state are initially admitted to the CCU, we and others feel that such patients should be removed from the CCU and placed in a separate unit (shock room or Intensive Care Unit). Even if they are transferred to an ICU the personnel most familiar with acute coronary disease will be intensively engaged in their care. Some hospitals will not have a room with special equipment for cardiogenic shock, and such patients are placed in the ICU. In any event they are so ill and require so much attention that they should be away from patients with uncomplicated myocardial infarctions.

Blood pressure is the net result of an adequate cardiac output, peripheral resistance and the capacitance of blood vessels. In acute myocardial infarction there is a reduction in blood pressure because of damage to the myocardium. This may be brief or prolonged depending on the extent of myocardial involvement and the compensatory changes which may take place. Alterations in blood pressure must be interpreted as one sign of the changes in a hemodynamic system, which with other variables must be integrated into the clinical picture.

Etiology

The mechanism of shock due to acute myocardial infarction is incompletely understood. The syndrome is associated with damage to the myocardium but no simple equation can be made between the degree of damage and the severity of shock. Shock due to myocardial infarction is associated with a diminished cardiac output. However, other complications of AMI are often associated with a profound reduction in cardiac output without shock, for example, extremes of slow and fast heart rates and congestive heart failure.

Autopsied patients who have died in shock show that the myocardial infarction is usually extensive. Hence, it is often inferred that all patients in shock have extensive infarction. Autopsies on patients who have died from recurrent arrhythmia or congestive heart failure frequently reveal extensive infarction even though shock did not dominate the clinical picture. Very little is actually known about the shock state in man during acute myocardial infarction. The available information indicates that the cardiac output is markedly reduced, the peripheral vascular resistance is usually high, but may be normal or low, and the total circulating blood volume is reduced. Perfusion of the coronary circulation is greatly reduced. Much research in man will be needed before the complete clinical picture of cardiogenic shock is understood.

The mortality rate in patients with acute myocardial infarction and shock is quite high, most authors reporting 80 percent; some reporting 100 percent. Studies reporting a dramatic lowering of the mortality rate in shock patients are misleading in that they probably include simple cases of hypotension without profound shock.

Clinical Assessment

The patient's blood pressure should be taken immediately upon admission to the CCU and as frequently as every 15 minutes for the next few hours, always by a competent member of the team. This important procedure is often relegated to a novice or an aid.

Automatic monitors presently available rely on the Koratkoff sounds. They record blood pressure every 15 minutes or more frequently, and display the results in lighted numbers. We have no experience with this machine but theoretically, at least, it should be useful.

Most patients who are normotensive prior to their infarcts have a transient fall in blood pressure from 10-30 mm Hg systolic to 5-10 mm Hg diastolic. The pressure returns to pre-infarction levels as the myocardium compensates, usually by the third hospital day. Sometimes the blood pressure falls to levels of 70 mm Hg systolic and 40 mm Hg diastolic, and remains so for many days to weeks with no apparent deleterious effect.

Acute myocardial infarction has a variable effect on the hypertensive patient. About one-third of hypertensive patients become normotensive after infarction; the remaining two-thirds return to hypertensive levels after a transient fall in blood pressure. Previously hypertensive patients may remain normotensive for as long as 2 years after infarction. Reliance on absolute numbers leads to serious errors in the acute stage. The severely hypertensive patient may be in shock with a blood pressure which otherwise would be considered normal. The level of the blood pressure should always be integrated into the clinical picture and previous history.

The clinical assessment of the shock state is difficult and in assessing any patient one must consider the following clinical findings.

1. *Hypotension* (no peripheral pulse or very low blood pressure by the cuff method).
2. *Decreased urine output* (failure to perfuse the kidney).
3. *Cold, clammy skin* (failure to perfuse the skin).
4. *Mental torpor* (failure to perfuse the brain).

When all four findings are present, the patient is unequivocally in shock. If only two are present the shock state is not as severe. The difficulties in evaluation and classification are apparent, as there are gradations of all of these parameters which should be evaluated as an indication of the presence or absence of shock in everyone with acute myocardial infarction.

When the above physical signs are present and have persisted for more than a few hours, the patient's situation is critical and a good outcome is unlikely. It is frequently stated that, as long as the patient produces a urine flow of one to two cc per minute. he is not in serious shock, and it is probable that he is not in serious shock if he has detectable peripheral blood pressure. When one is estimating the blood pressure in a patient with shock, the only guideline available is the peripheral blood pressure. The fact that the patient has no detectable blood pressure by the cuff method is of dire significance, regardless of whether or not one can feel his femoral pulse or palpate the carotid pulsations.

1. *The blood pressure:* As indicated above, the absence of the peripheral blood pressure, as measured by the sphygmomanometer cuff, indicates an ominous prognosis. This is not always so and measurements of direct arterial pressure by direct puncture of the artery and estimation of the pressure in the central aortic position (central aortic pressure) may occasionally reveal levels of blood pressure in the central aorta which are quite high, even when no detectable peripheral pulses are discernible. It is not uncommon, for example, to record a blood pressure in the central aorta of 70/40 in the absence of a peripheral pulse. The discrepancy between the cuff pressure and the central aortic pressure is thought to be due to an extremely high peripheral resistance which involves the medium-sized arteries. This is of some importance because we feel that vasopressor agents are not indicated unless the mean central aortic pressure is below 60 mm Hg. A knowledge of the central aortic pressure is important because the indiscriminate use of vasopressor agents may precipitate ventricular fibrillation. It is generally estimated that a mean blood pressure in the central aortic position of 60 mm Hg is necessary to perfuse the kidney and the coronary arteries. We feel that as long as the central aortic pressure is above this level, it is not necessary and, perhaps, is dangerous to give vasopressor agents. If the pressure is below this level, vasopressor agents need to be given.

What is essentially being stated above is that, in the absence of the other manifestations of shock, the patient whose peripheral blood pressure is low does not necessarily have a very bad prognosis. One does not need to treat levels of peripheral blood pressure (cuff method) in the range of 60 to 70 mm Hg systolic by vasopressor agents in the absence of other signs of shock.

2. *Urine output* in cardiogenic shock is proportional to glomerular filtration rate (GFR) which is related to cardiac output. In the absence of intrinsic renal disease (BUN less than 20) a urine flow of 1.0 cc/minute indicates adequate renal perfusion. As long as urine is produced in such quantities nothing need be done about elevating cuff pressure or blood pressure. Glomerular filtration continues with maintenance of a mean arterial pressure of 60 mm Hg, but below this level urine formation stops. By inference, a patient with no recordable peripheral blood pressure who continues to produce urine has a mean aortic pressure well above 60 mm Hg. The kidney in shock fails to excrete sodium. Levels below 30mEq/liter of urine are noted. This should be taken into consideration when replacing fluids. The administration of saline to expand blood volume should be questioned under these circumstances as the patient can be thrown into congestive heart failure.

3. *Cold and clammy skin* signifies high peripheral *resistance.* Peripheral resistance must be measured indirectly and relies on the accuracy of two parameters derived with difficulty, the cardiac output and blood pressure. The measurement of *cardiac output* in the shock state as in other low output situations is very inaccurate. Indirect measurements using the Fick principle are difficult because of the inaccuracy of measuring oxygen consumption in a hyperventilating and uncooperative patient. Direct measurements with dye dilution techniques are equally inaccurate because of the error in mathematically measuring the area beneath a splayed-out curve. Variation of as much as 25 percent can be recorded in sequential measurements of cardiac output, which makes assessment of treatment difficult. The measurement of blood pressure is easier to record, but here again variations of as much as 30 mm Hg exist between the central aorta and radial artery. Peripheral resistance is a derived measurement and clinically is correlated with cold and clammy skin. Most cases of shock due to myocardial infarct are associated with high peripheral resistance. Some cases, however, fail to elevate resistance, a failure of compensatory mechanism. The expression of peripheral resistance is related to the total resistance. This neglects consideration of the variable and selective resistances from one organ to another. Cold and clammy extremities are a sign of high peripheral resistance. Further increments of resistance are neither useful nor safe. The advocates of

pressor amines suggest that the efficacy of these drugs is related to the enhancement of cardiac output or to the adjustment of compensatory mechanisms to elevate peripheral resistance.

4. *Mental torpor.* The significance of confusion, agitation, and obstreperous personality due to cerebral anoxia have been misinterpreted for many years. The sudden appearance of a personality change or a clouded sensorium indicates a decrease in cardiac output. Unfortunately no correlation can be made between personality change and cardiac output as can be made with urine production and blood pressure. In the low cardiac output state of advanced mitral stenosis, "mitral madness" indicates cardiac outputs below 2 liters/minute. Mental torpor is a clear indication that vital central nervous system centers are not being perfused with oxygenated blood. The cardiac output is probably of the order of 2 liters/minute or less.

Management of the Hypotensive Patient

No specific therapy is available; however, vital functions listed below must be monitored. These will be discussed in sequence. Correction of specific abnormalities have sometimes been associated with a favorable outcome.

MONITOR	VITAL FUNCTION
Central venous pressure	Blood volume
Urine flow (Foley catheter)	Renal blood flow
Arterial gas analysis	Electrolyte stability and oxygen transport
Central aortic pressure	Blood pressure (central)
Respiration with a respirator and ventilometer	Ventilation and oxygenation

CENTRAL VENOUS PRESSURE (CVP)

Central venous pressure (CVP) may be recorded by introducing a polyethylene tubing through a basillic vein, advancing it intrathoracically and attaching it to a water manometer (Fig. 1). Entrance into the thoracic cavity is heralded by the prompt drop in pressure on inspiration, and elevation with expiration. The superior vena cava is desirable but any vein within the thoracic cavity is equally suitable. When the patient is being ventilated by positive pressure machines, this fluctuation in the central venous pressure is reversed. For those

BEDSIDE   CENTRAL   VENOUS   PRESSURE

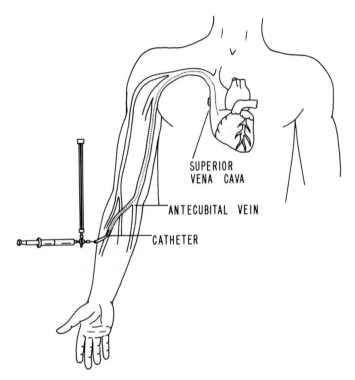

SUPERIOR
VENA CAVA

ANTECUBITAL VEIN

CATHETER

Fig. 1. A method of estimating central venous pressure. A polyethylene catheter is threaded through a basilic vein to the level of the left atrium and connected to a 3-way stopcock with a water manometer. CVP is read directly from the manometer when the zero point of reference is at the level of the left atrium.

who are more experienced, the CVP may be obtained by subclavian vein puncture. The subclavian vein is a fixed landmark and immediately available when other peripheral veins are difficult to puncture. This procedure should not be taken lightly by the uninitiated but for those with some degree of proficiency it is a safe technique.

The zero point of reference is on a level with the left atrium. The normal CVP ranges between 2 and 10 cm H_2O. Central venous pressure above 12 cm H_2O is evidence of an overloaded circulation and suggests congestive heart failure. A rapidly acting digitalis preparation should be given. If the CVP is below 2 cm H_2O or is unrecordable (zero), it may be inferred that the patient is suffering from hypovolemia. Volume may be cautiously replaced with plasma, dextran, or saline (fluid challenge). However, constant observation of the CVP must be made during infusion. Any sudden rise in the venous pressure should curtail "volume expansion." The patient with an apparently normal or low CVP should probably have the benefit of volume expansion prior to the institution of any other therapy. Fluid is introduced in units of 250 cc given over 5 to 10 minutes. A rise of CVP of more than 5 mm as a result of this "fluid push" is an indication to cease the administration of the fluid. One to three liters of D/W are frequently administered to the hypotensive patient with markedly beneficial results.

Perhaps the full realization of the concept of diminished blood volume and the use of the CVP is the most important aspect of the management of the hypotensive patient. Certainly this aspect of the clinical problem must be attended to before any vasopressors are given. It is surprising how often the hypotensive patient will become normotensive as a result of the above procedure, and the true shock state averted. Some notion of this mechanism is shown in Fig. 2.

RENAL BLOOD FLOW AND URINE FLOW

Since much information about the central circulation is gained from renal hemodynamics, it is imperative to record urine flow accurately. The patient in shock is usually unable to cooperate enough to void when desired so that the use of an indwelling catheter is justified. The catheter is connected to a graduated plastic container. Urine flow is monitored at half-hourly intervals at first, and when therapy appears to be beneficial at hourly intervals. When indwelling catheters are used for reasons other than the accurate recording of urine flow, the 3-way Foley for constant bladder irrigation is employed.

ARTERIAL GAS ANALYSIS

Arterial blood for gas analysis should be drawn from all hypotensive patients. The "blood gases" will give important information in two areas: the oxygen tension and saturation on the one hand, and the pH, PCO_2, and bicarbonate on the other. A discussion of oxygen and pulmonary ventilation is given below. The patient in shock is with rare exception in metabolic acidosis. It is necessary to assess the severity of acidosis, the degree of respiratory compensation, and the concomitant level of oxygen tension before any therapeutic program can be instituted. There is no reason for gas analysis to be unavail-

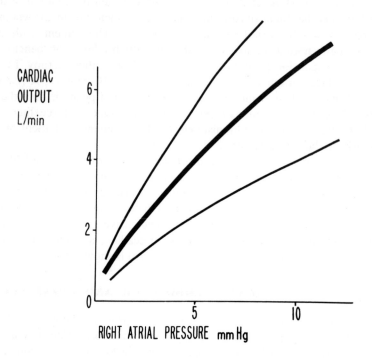

Fig. 2. The above diagram indicates the relationship between right atrial or central venous pressure and cardiac output. The heavy middle line shows that the cardiac output is directly related to right atrial pressure. This curve is the basis for the use of the fluid "push" for managing patients with lowered cardiac output. It is of interest to note that the lower line indicating the curve for patients with diminished cardiac output also shows a response to fluid loads. The upper line shows the effect of adrenergic response.

able in the modern hospital. Specimens of arterial blood are collected by puncture of the femoral artery with a 20-gauge needle attached to a heparinized syringe. The specimen should be sealed and analyzed immediately. If this is not feasible it should be refrigerated, since pH decreases at room temperature. When indicated, treatment should be promptly instituted by infusing $NaHCO_3$ intravenously. Total bicarbonate deficit is calculated as follows:

(Normal HCO_3 in mEq/liter — observed HCO_3 in mEq/liter)
$\times$ (body wt in kg $\times$ 20%)

The bicarbonate may be given as a bolus injection of 44 mEq at a time and subsequent determinations of pH made to estimate the degree of improvement. Overcorrecting acidosis represents little hazard. The transient metabolic alkalosis is soon corrected by hyperventilation and by the continuing abnormal metabolic process which produces acid.

Alkalosis in shock is always respiratory in origin and produced by hyperventilation owing to severe hypoxemia. Correction of hypoxemia is essential, and the administration of oxygen by nasal cannula is not always effective in the presence of shock. Assisted ventilation is required, and often controlled ventilation is necessary. No attempt can be made at the correction of pH abnormalities or the institution of assisted ventilation without arterial gas analysis. To do so without these crucial tests would be a misguided effort.

The frequency of severe respiratory alkalosis is striking as shown in the following data from St. Vincent's Hospital (Table 1).

TABLE 1. *Incidence of Blood Gas Abnormalities*

Hypoxemia (50-70 mm Hg)	342	22.8%
Extreme Hypoxemia (under 50 mm Hg)	259	17.3%
Alkalosis, Respiratory	657	43.8%
Alkalosis, Metabolic	124	8.3%
Acidosis, Respiratory	174	11.6%
Acidosis, Metabolic	112	7.4%
Within Normal Limits	134	8.9%
Total Studies	1500	

CONTROLLED VENTILATION IN SHOCK

The patient in severe shock frequently cannot be oxygenated by mask oxygen. Positive pressure mask oxygen is occasionally inadequate and endotracheal or nasotracheal intubation is necessary with the tracheal tube connected to a ventilating device, preferably a volume cycle respirator.

The patient must be intubated with a *cuffed* endotracheal tube. This is a simple procedure, well-tolerated, and essential to the proper delivery of oxygen: A respirometer must be available and used frequently. Unfortunately, the prescription of tidal volumes is not as accurate as one could desire. The error in ventilatory machines is enormous. The tidal volume must be checked with a respirometer every 15 minutes when a patient is first connected to a ventilatory machine. The frequency of tidal volume assessment can be diminished after the machine has been calibrated to the patient. Arterial gas analysis must be obtained at 2-hour intervals until the proper tidal volume is reached. It is amazing to observe the incredibly high tidal volumes in hypoxic alkalotic patients who clinically appear to be breathing normally.

It has been our experience that some patients in shock due to myocardial infarction have a twofold defect. They are hypoxic and become alkalotic (respiratory) due to hyperventilation in an attempt to correct the oxygen defect. Secondly, shock produces metabolic acidosis which depletes the bicarbonate reserve. There is now a very complex situation consisting of mixed respiratory alkalosis and metabolic acidosis. The following should then be done more or less simultaneously.

1. Oxygen given to raise Po_2 and prevent tissue anoxia.
2. Bicarbonate reserves increased by giving bicarbonate intravenously.
3. Controlled ventilation (reducing the tidal volume) to allow the Pco_2 to rise.

Small doses of demerol (5 mg i.v.) and phenergan (10 mg i.v.) are given every hour to help the patient who has trouble tolerating the cuffed endotracheal tube.

There is some apprehension about administration of positive pressure oxygen as this may decrease the flow of blood to the right ventricle and diminish cardiac output. If this happens under the circumstances of severe shock, the lowering is modest and is a small price to pay for a higher Po_2.

CENTRAL AORTIC PRESSURE

Using the Seldinger technique a peripheral artery, preferably the femoral, should be catheterized and connected to a strain gauge manometer. The character of the pulse pressure curve provides useful information. The systolic and mean arterial pressures are accurately measured. Extremes of peripheral resistance can be diagnosed without cumbersome determination of cardiac output (which is notoriously inaccurate at low levels). The first derivative of the upslope (DP/DT) can be measured, and if severely impaired may be treated with inotropic agents. Admittedly, direct arterial measurements require a great deal of equipment and attendants. If available, it should be used for all patients in shock (Fig. 3).

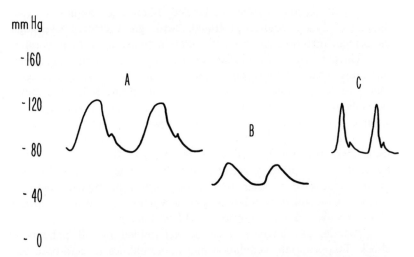

Fig. 3. Direct arterial pulse tracings. Normally arterial pressure rapidly rises to systolic levels and, following closure of the aortic valve marked by the dicrotic notch, falls gradually to diastolic levels (A). Decreased cardiac output usually leads to a fall in both systolic and diastolic pressure (B). Decreased stroke output together with marked increase in peripheral resistance results in a very rapid pressure rise in systole followed by a rapid fall to diastolic levels. Mean arterial pressure is very close to diastolic levels (C).

METABOLIC CHANGES IN SHOCK

The inadequate circulation (low cardiac output) in shock leads to tissue hypoxia. There is inadequate perfusion of the brain, lungs, kidneys, muscles, and other vital organs which leads to metabolic acidosis. As hypoxia becomes marked, lactic acidosis sets in and is apparently irreversible because of a failure to convert pyruvate to carbon dioxide and water. Inadequate cardiac output then precipitates a vicious cycle—hypoxemia—hypoxia—poor tissue perfusion—deteriorating tissue and organ function—metabolic acidosis—lactic acidosis—and the total effect on the myocardium is a further diminution of cardiac output. Arrhythmias which are notoriously difficult to treat are then produced.

SUMMARY OF MANAGEMENT

Every patient in shock should be challenged by a fluid load while central venous pressure and urine flow are monitored. Reliance on dye-dilution and radioactive labeled dilution techniques for estimation of blood volume is fraught with great error. Physiologic assessment including the central venous pressure appears preferable.

The correction of acidosis is crucial. This may require the generous prescription of bicarbonate. Acidosis does not remain corrected unless renal function is adequate. Perfusion of the kidneys requires not only an adequate blood pressure but an effective circulating blood volume. The elevation of base reserve, however, is not the total solution to the problem. Hyperventilation which accompanies shock is usually not reversed by correction of acidosis. The hyperventilation appears to be a primary defect in the shock state and must be adequately controlled in order to effectively restore permanent acid-base balance. Controlled ventilation with a volume cycled respirator is almost always required to restore acid-base balance.

Arterial gas analysis must be determined on all patients in shock. Inappropriate ventilation and abnormalities in acid-base balance must be corrected if they are present.

VASOPRESSOR AGENTS

We feel strongly that there is no room for the prescription of pressor drugs for shock in acute myocardial infarction until the preceding measurements of vital function are assessed and appropriately treated.

Once the pH is corrected, ventilation instituted, and CVP controlled, there remains a group of patients who still remain in shock. Subsequent therapy in these cases is controversial. Most investigators and clinicians agree that beta-mimetic drugs such as levophed have not altered the mortality of cardiogenic shock and are probably contraindicated in high resistance states. The alternative choice of therapy, theoretically at least, is a drug such as isoproterenol which increases stroke output (beta mimetic) and decreases peripheral resistance (alpha blocker). The difficulty with isoproterenol is that it possesses marked chronotropic properties which produce serious tachycardia. The control of peripheral resistance is difficult. Another drug, yet unavailable, is needed to selectively block the chronotropic properties of isoproterenol. Another alternative is a combination of drugs such as neosynephrine or vasoxyl, alpha mimetic drugs, and phenoxybenzamine (Dibenzyline), an alpha blocker. There is no substantial experience to indicate that one vasopressor agent is preferable to another.

Prescription of pressor amines is not the panacea it was once considered. Rather than improve the circulation, restoration of "normal" blood pressure may result in a decreased cardiac output and ventricular fibrillation.

Hypotension without shock is a very thorny problem in acute myocardial infarction. If the patient is warm, clear headed, and producing urine, the blood pressure is not treated, no matter what the cuff pressure reading. It is extremely difficult to convince one's colleagues to refrain from action and to withhold levophed in these circumstances. The need to do something should be replaced by vigorous attention to pH, hypoxemia, and central venous pressure. To refrain from prescribing vasopressors is not equated with doing nothing. Actually, "doing nothing" requires more work because the patient must be monitored more carefully and closely. The critical blood pressure in the central aortic area is approximately 60 mm Hg mean (mean B.P. = two-thirds of systolic pressure). As long as mean B.P. is 60 or more, we do not give vasopressors.

OTHER DRUGS

There is no data to indicate that digitalis is of any benefit in this situation. The use of corticosteroids is controversial, although probably not harmful.

MECHANICAL DEVICES

Mechanical devices such as counter pulsation, assisted circulation, and mechanical hearts are still in the developmental state.

References

Elliott, W. C., and Gorlin, R. Isoproterenol in treatment of heart disease. J.A.M.A., 197:315, 1966.

Gunnar, R. M., Loeb, H. S., Pietras, R. J., and Tobin, J. R. Hemodynamic measurements in a coronary care unit. Prog. Cardiovasc. Dis., 11:29, 1968.

Mackenzie, G. J., et al. Circulatory and respiratory studies in myocardial infarction and cardiogenic shock. Lancet, 2:825, 1964.

Soroff, H. S., Giron, F., Ruiz, U., Birtwell, W. C., Hirsh, L. J. and Deterling, R. A. Physiologic support by heart action. New Eng. J. Med., 280:693, 1969.

Thomas, M., Malmcrona, R., and Shillingford, J. P. Circulatory changes associated with systemic hypotension in patients with acute myocardial infarction. Brit. Heart J., 28:108, 1966.

Weil, M. H., and Shubin, H. Shock following acute myocardial infarct: Current understanding of hemodynamic mechanisms. Prog. Cardiovasc. Dis., 11:1, 1968.

—————— and Shubin, H. Diagnosis and Treatment of Shock. Baltimore, The Williams & Wilkins Company, 1967.

—————— Shubin, H., Rosoff, L. Fluid repletion in circulatory shock. J.A.M.A., 192:84, 1965.

8

Cardiac Arrest
and Resuscitation

Cardiac arrest is the sudden cessation of effective circulation. This definition implies a sudden, unpredictable, and abrupt interruption of the heart function; not a gradual diminution of cardiac output as in congestive heart failure or shock. Cardiac arrest from any cause is tantamount to death unless immediately treated. It has been clearly demonstrated that cardiac arrest need not be a terminal event of life. In many cases it is completely reversible and with successful resuscitation, may be associated with functional life for a very long time. The first patient we successfully resuscitated from cardiac arrest and acute myocardial infarction (1961) is still living and well.

Causes of
Cardiac Arrest

Cardiac arrest is electrocardiographically represented by ventricular fibrillation or ventricular asystole. These arrhythmias usually appear abruptly but may be heralded by other arrhythmias such as frequent premature ventricular contractions, complete heart block, or varying degrees of second degree heart block. Idioventricular rhythm which is unable to sustain life is not considered a cause of cardiac arrest but rather a terminal event of congestive heart failure, shock, or other arrhythmias. Cardiac arrest is an electrical derangement and, theoretically, reversible.

Despite every effort to treat life-threatening arrhythmias, cardiac arrest continues to occur. Sudden cessation of effective heart beat and loss of cardiac output is due to either failure of impulse formation (cardiac standstill) or ineffective impulse formation (ventricular fibrillation). Patients with cardiac standstill are rarely resuscitated. Experience with cardiac monitoring has demonstrated that failure of impulse formation is uncommon in acute myocardial infarction. Over three-fourths of the episodes of cardiac arrest in patients with myocardial infarction are due to ventricular fibrillation. Ventricular fibrillation in myocardial infarction has been categorized as "primary," appearing without premonitory warning, and "secondary," appearing as an event during shock or congestive heart failure. Treatment of ventricular premature beats and ventricular tachycardia has decreased the incidence of primary ventricular fibrillation. While some physicians claim to have abolished ventricular fibrillation altogether, experience from most coronary care units suggests that this phenomenon still occurs. Most ventricular fibrillation (VF) occurs early in the course of acute myocardial infarction. If the Emergency Room of the hospital is seeing "early cases," more ventricular fibrillation will be seen than if admission is delayed.

The reversibility of cardiac arrest is proportional to the speed and skill of delivering effective therapy. While the prevention of cardiac arrest dominates the organization of the CCU, an effective system of treating cardiac arrest must be available.

Diagnosis of Cardiac Arrest

Diagnosis of cardiac arrest may be based on definitive or presumptive evidence. Definitive diagnosis is made by demonstrating ventricular fibrillation or ventricular asystole on a cardiac monitor or on electrocardiographic paper. The diagnosis is readily established in a patient who is attached to a monitor and the oscilloscopic representation of fatal ventricular arrhythmia may be recorded on electrocardiographic paper within seconds. However, the patient may not be connected to a monitor or the monitor may be malfunctioning. In this case the presumptive diagnosis of cardiac arrest may then be made on the following clinical criteria:

1. Convulsion. A tonic-clonic seizure is frequently associated with heart block. The Adams-Stokes syndrome in the setting of acute heart disease is good evidence of the abrupt cessation of effective heart beat due either to ventricular fibrillation or asystole. Treatment is directed toward restoration of heart beat and not toward control of the convulsion. When a patient with acute myocardial infarction suffers a convulsive seizure he should be defibrillated immediately. No time should be lost in establishing an electrocardiographic diagnosis: Defibrillate immediately.

2. Apnea. Continued apnea in an unconscious patient heralds cardiovascular collapse. Cheyne-Stokes respiration may be associated with prolonged periods of apnea but rarely lasts over 20 seconds. The patient with Cheyne-Stokes respiration, if unconscious, can usually be aroused. The pulse is palpable during the apneic periods. Apnea for more than 20 seconds calls for immediate action. Sudden gasping respiration in a patient who previously was breathing normally should be included under apnea as all respiration soon ceases if cardiac arrest has occurred.

3. Absent pulses. The abrupt cessation of pulses should be considered a manifestation of cardiac arrest until proven otherwise. Rapid tachycardia may make the pulse feeble and difficult to palpate but cardiac sounds are usually audible. When a radial pulse is lost an attempt should be made to palpate the femoral or carotid pulsation. Even with extremely low cardiac output the femoral pulse is usually palpable. The carotid pulse should be avoided so as not to compromise the cerebral circulation. Asystole may be precipitated by carotid sinus pressure.

4. Absent heart sounds. Heart sounds in acute myocardial infarction may become very feeble. They are muffled by emphysema and obesity. When sounds previously audible suddenly disappear, cardiac arrest should be the first consideration. In all patients with feeble sounds, the location of the point of maximal impulse should be marked upon admission to the CCU with a skin pencil as a point of future reference.

5. *Dilation of the pupils.* This is a late sign of cardiac arrest and subject to considerable variability. The presence of dilated pupils indicates that cardiac arrest has been present for at least 30 seconds and probably for more than 60 seconds. However, with good resuscitation dilated pupils will return to normal size. This does not preclude total recovery.

Resuscitation

Treatment of cardiac arrest should be instituted whenever a presumptive diagnosis is made and should not be delayed for a definitive diagnosis. Clinically, the patient with cardiac arrest from any cause presents simultaneously the features of absent pulse, blood pressure, and respiration. Successful resuscitation requires a restoration of all three abnormalities. These will be discussed separately but at the bedside all are treated concurrently, and treatment often overlaps.

1. *Absent pulse.* Since most cases of cardiac arrest are due to ventricular fibrillation, electric defibrillation should be performed when presumptive evidence of cardiac arrest is present and before an electrocardiogram is obtained. Defibrillation of the patient with ventricular standstill does no harm. The defibrillator must be instantly available at all times in the coronary care unit. Prompt defibrillation often eliminates the necessity of circulatory and respiratory support. Should the patient not respond immediately to ventricular defibrillation he must be supported with closed chest cardiac massage and ventilation until a specific diagnosis and evaluation of the problem is made.

2. *Apnea.* The apneic patient must have his ventilation supported. Most resuscitative failures in the treatment of cardiac arrest result from an inability to maintain ventilation because of the resistance of the anoxic myocardium to defibrillation.

The most convenient and least time-consuming method of ventilatory support is the Ambu-type bag with oxygen administration (Fig. 1). This is superior to mouth-to-mouth insufflation and certainly more esthetic. The patient's neck should be extended and the jaw pulled up. An oral airway should then be inserted to prevent the tongue from occluding the laryngeal orifice. The Ambu bag is next fitted snugly over the patient's face so that it seals the nose and mouth. By simply compressing the Ambu bag with the hand at a rate

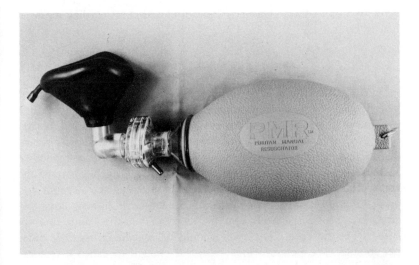

Fig. 1. Self inflating breathing bag with face mask. Ventilation may be performed by snuggly applying the face mask over the nose and mouth and periodically squeezing the bag. Oxygen may be administered by attaching an oxygen catheter to the side arm. A one-way valve is provided to prevent rebreathing expired air.

of 20 times per minute, most patients who are apneic can be ventilated. An oxygen catheter can be connected to the bag to deliver higher oxygen tension than room air.

If an experienced physician is present, intubation with a cuffed endotracheal tube may be attempted. Ventilation with the Ambu bag is now made much more effective. Assisted or controlled ventilation with a pressure- or volume-cycled respirator may be substituted for the Ambu bag. Tracheostomy has no place in the treatment of apnea due to cardiac arrest. This is a difficult and time-consuming procedure in the best hands. After the patient is ventilated and oxygenation is improved—indicated by the appearance of the skin and mucous membranes—further attempts to defibrillate the patient may be made, if necessary.

3. Loss of circulation. The abrupt loss of pulses or blood pressure indicates no effective circulation. Until the patient can be defibrillated or until specific medications can be administered which enhance the effectiveness of defibrillation, the circulation must be assisted. Opening the chest and manually massaging the heart may produce an effective circulation but there is rarely a permanent survivor by this method. The technique of closed-chest cardiac massage is used exclusively.

TECHNIQUE OF CLOSED-CHEST MASSAGE

The patient must be placed on a bed board or a firm stretcher. The floor is a poor substitute because it is very difficult to attend a patient on one's hands and knees. The heel of one hand is placed over the lower one-third of the sternum above the xiphoid process and the other hand placed on top of it. Vertical pressure is applied so as to depress the sternum a distance of 1.5 to 2.0 inches toward the spine. This technique compresses the heart between the sternum and spine forcing blood into the systemic circulation. Following compression, pressure is released from the sternum but the hands are not lifted from the chest. The cycle should be repeated about 60 times per minute. The pressure must be great enough to cause a femoral pulse which must be continuously monitored. This technique is very demanding and fatiguing. Whenever possible a portable compressor should be used. It not only keeps cardiac massage constant but also frees an additional hand to lend assistance elsewhere. A suitable inexpensive model is shown in Figure 2. Mechanical chest compressors, air driven or electrically driven, are frequently clumsy to apply and are no more effective than manual compression.

The complications of closed-chest massage include fractured ribs, lacerated liver, and pneumothorax. The enthusiastic house staff physician is more likely to be vigorous with pressure than the predictable hand mechanical compressor. The treatment of fractured ribs represents little difficulty; they heal with no specific therapy. Strapping the chest is contraindicated so that ventilation will not be impaired. Pneumothorax is rarely extensive. If it represents more than 20 percent of the lung area as seen on a conventional roentgenogram, a chest tube should be inserted and connected to underwater drainage. During resuscitation the physician must always keep in mind the possibility of developing a tension pneumothorax, and repeatedly examine the patient for this. Laceration of the liver represents the most serious complication and uniformly leads to death from exsanguination. Fortunately it is a rare complication and has not been seen since the early days of closed-chest massage. Transfusions may be helpful but surgery is interdicted by the very nature of the underlying cardiac arrest.

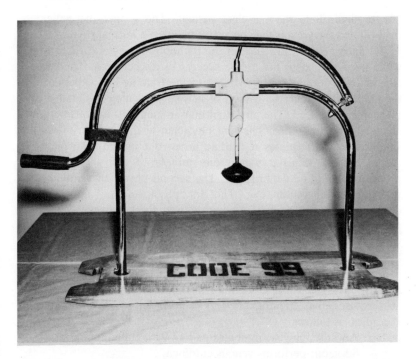

Fig. 2. A simple device for maintaining closed-chest cardiac massage. The board is placed under the patient and the aluminum rod fit into place. A single operator can maintain closed-chest massage for long periods of time without experiencing fatigue.

PREPAREDNESS

It should be emphasized that there are no one-two-three steps to the treatment of cardiac arrest. The exact order of resuscitation depends on the number of personnel available. Ventilation and closed chest massage usually require two individuals. The first person on the scene should prepare for defibrillation. Another should obtain an electrocardiogram and establish a route for the administration of intravenous fluid. Since most cases of cardiac arrest occur within the first few hospital days, an indwelling intravenous catheter or scalp vein needle is inserted in all cases of acute myocardial infarction and maintained while the patient is in the CCU. When a physician or nurse is present at the moment of ventricular fibrillation, DC defibrillation can be done within a few seconds. One should not hesitate to defibrillate the pulseless patient. The sooner the patient is defibrillated the greater the chance of restoring a normal rhythm.

Fundamental knowledge of the pathophysiology of cardiac arrest, while necessary, does not assure success in resuscitation. The success rate of resuscitation is proportional to the training and experience of the staff. There must be a plan of action, meticulously detailed and frequently practiced. The physician may in many institutions be interchanged with the nurse. The first physician at the scene assesses the situation and determines if cardiac arrest did indeed take place. If cardiac arrest occurred within one minute of arrival, the patient promptly should be defibrillated. The second physician ventilates the patient with an Ambu bag. The first physician may now attempt defibrillation again or continue with closed-chest massage. The third physician obtains a 12-lead electrocardiogram, and provides an intravenous route of drug administration if one is not already available. He should spell the first physician at closed-chest cardiac massage. The cause of cardiac arrest should be determined and appropriate therapy instituted. Not more than three people are usually required at a resuscitative attempt, but others may help to institute specific therapies, as follows:

Anesthesiologist: intubates patient with cuffed tube;

Surgeon: performs venous cutdown;

Oxygen therapist: provides appropriate equipment;

Nurse: prepares necessary drugs for administration; dispenses medicine from the crash cart; brings the defibrillator to the bedside, plugs it in, adjusts the electrical dose and coats the paddles with electrode jelly. This should be done *while* the first physician is assessing the patient for cardiac arrest and not after his diagnosis is made. Every second is precious.

CARDIAC RHYTHMS ENCOUNTERED AFTER DEFIBRILLATION AND THEIR MANAGEMENT

1. Sinus rhythm with an adequate blood pressure. This represents complete success in treatment of cardiac arrest. Further treatment is indicated only if the precipitating event is documented. Prophylactic antiarrhythmic agents are generally not indicated since most are negatively inotropic.

2. Asystole. Absolute pacemaker failure may follow upon defibrillation. Pacemaker tissue may be stimulated with intracardiac epinephrine. If an intravenous route is readily available, epinephrine may be administered directly. The dose of epinephrine is 3 to 5 cc of a 1:10,000 solution. This is obtained by diluting one cc of the usually available 1:1,000 solution with 9 cc of sterile saline. After injection, cardiac massage must be maintained until the medication reaches the coronary circulation. If an intravenous route is not immediately available, then epinephrine should be introduced through an intracardiac needle. Care should be exercised to administer epinephrine into a ventricular cavity and not the ventricular myocardium. Aspiration of blood indicates that the needle is in a ventricular chamber. Myocardial injection of epinephrine may produce irreversible ventricular fibrillation. If pacemaker tissue is stimulated by epinephrine, it may be followed by the administration of isoproterenol (Isuprel). The dose of Isuprel is usually arrived at by trial. To one liter of dextrose solution is added 5 ampules of Isuprel (1 mg). This makes a solution of 1 μg per ml which can be titrated until an effective response is achieved. Epinephrine is probably the most effective drug in restoring pacemaker function. However, its continued use is toxic to the myocardium. In contrast to epinephrine, Isuprel has a potent effect as a peripheral vasodilator. If an effective heart beat is maintained by infusing Isuprel, a pressor amine may be required to maintain an effective blood pressure.

A *transvenous* pacemaker is sometimes useful but its insertion under the circumstances of cardiac arrest is a harrowing experience. For this reason its prophylactic insertion is recommended in those conditions which are frequently associated with cardiac arrest and asystole. Percutaneous introduction of an electric pacemaker through the precordium and directly into the myocardium has been attempted by us in 15 consecutive cases of asystole. There have been no survivors.

3. Heart block with recurrent ventricular fibrillation. The objective of treatment in this disorder is to stimulate the highest pacemaker. The "irritable focus" should not be suppressed with procainamide, (Pronestyl) or quinidine with resultant asystole. Actually the "irritable focus" may be the only pacemaker available. The mechanism of recurrent ventricular fibrillation in the setting of heart block is bradycardia. Isuprel is the treatment of choice (*vide supra*) until a transvenous pacemaker can be inserted. Once an effective rate of 50 or 60 beats per minute is established with an adequate blood pressure, the heart block disappears and the administration of Isuprel can be tapered off. Atropine sulfate may have a beneficial result in some patients with heart block. The dose is 2 mg intravenously. The vagolytic effect of atropine is usually complete with this dose, and higher doses will not accelerate the heart rate any further. Low doses of atropine, 0.4 mg (grain 1/150), have no effect under situations of cardiac arrest.

4. *For recurrent ventricular tachycardia* the management consists of proper ventilatory care and drug treatment. Bretylium tosylate (100 mg I.V. or 300 mg I.M.) is given "stat" and q. 6-8 hrs. This drug will probably replace lidocaine which is in wide current use for ventricular tachycardia. The dose of lidocaine is a bolus of 25 mg followed by a continuous I.V. drip of lidocaine 500 mg in 500 cc. The speed of administration is regulated to obtain the desired effect. Occasionally, when the above fail, pacing the myocardium via a transvenous pacemaker is effective. (See also chapter 5, p. 123.)

CIRCULATORY SUPPORT

When the arrhythmias which precipitated cardiac arrest or resulted from it have been controlled, attention must then be directed to supporting the circulation. This entails treatment of the blood pressure. Acidosis develops very rapidly after cardiac arrest, no matter how brief. Blood pH must be completely and promptly corrected. This correction alone may be enough to elevate blood pressure. If a resuscitative effort lasts more than a few moments, the most available member of the team should arrange for intravenous therapy by performing a "cut down" on a vein. A solution of 5 percent sodium bicarbonate should be attached and freely prescribed throughout a resuscitative procedure. Other agents such as THAM (tris-hydroxy-aminomethane) are not as effective in treating acidosis. Arterial gas analysis, especially arterial pH, should be determined, if possible, to assess the effectiveness of therapy.

If the blood pressure continues to be low after the restoration of rhythm and acid-base equilibrium, ventilatory assistance must be considered. Arterial oxygen tension must be determined. Abnormally low oxygen tensions which are commonly found after cardiac arrest should be corrected with a volume-cycled respirator. A normal tidal volume effectively delivered for several minutes causes prompt correction of hypoxemia and frequently results in an elevation of the blood pressure. Pressure-cycled machines are not as effective during cardiac arrest. The high airway resistance, mucous secretions, and external cardiac massage cause the respirator to discharge without delivering an adequate tidal volume. Volume-cycled respirators are preferred.

There has been a tendency to give vasopressor agents to patients who have low blood pressure. Because of the dangers of restarting or initiating ventricular fibrillation with vasopressors, we have become very cautious in prescribing them.

We suggest that the patients with low blood pressure or shock after a resuscitation be further managed as described in the section on shock, with emphasis on monitoring the central venous and central aortic pressure. Much more can be accomplished in raising blood pressure via fluid replacement than with vasopressors. We feel that no vasopressor should be given without continued monitoring of CVP and aortic pressure.

COMA FOLLOWING RESUSCITATION FROM VENTRICULAR FIBRILLATION

Once there is spontaneous heartbeat, pulse and blood pressure, and spontaneous respirations, the patient usually regains consciousness. However, this is not always so, and we have had patients remain unconscious for as long as 48 hours and ultimately make a complete recovery.

RESPIRATORY SUPPORT

Besides restoring circulation, the most important therapy for cardiac arrest is adequate ventilation. In some cases ventilation eclipses circulation in its importance because many arrhythmias are refractory to therapy while hypoxia and derangements of pH persist. In the apneic unconscious patient the problems of airway management are multiplied. Mouth-to-mouth resuscitation has been a long-established practice. This therapy requires a great deal of dedication and selflessness and has generally been abandoned for the more popular "S"-shaped Guedel oropharyngeal tube (Safar)* or the mask and self-inflating bag (Ambu). The patient's neck is hyperextended to keep the oropharynx patent. A Safar tube similar to an oropharyngeal airway is inserted in the mouth. A mouthpiece is provided which acts as a mask. The patient may be ventilated in this manner until more suitable equipment can be provided. A more efficient and less cumbersome tool for providing ventilation is the Ambu bag. In a similar fashion the head is hyperextended and an oropharyngeal airway is

---

* The "S" oropharyngeal tube is sold by Johnson and Johnson Company as "Resusitube."

inserted to keep the tongue forward. The mask of the apparatus is applied snugly over the nose and mouth. Ventilation is provided by squeezing the bag intermittently. Higher concentrations of oxygen can be delivered by connecting an ordinary oxygen catheter to the bag. The Ambu bag is equipped with a one-way valve so that rebreathing is prevented. In this manner ventilation can be provided almost indefinitely. The best method of ventilating the apneic patient is by using a volume-cycled respirator through a cuffed endotracheal tube. When this method is not readily available, the Ambu bag-type ventilation should be used.

The endotracheal tube is well tolerated. It must be remembered that when an endotracheal tube is in place the patient's natural defense of pulmonary infection may be disturbed. Tracheal suction must be performed with sterile catheters. It is imperative that sidearm escape holes be provided during aspiration so that the trachea and bronchi are not continuously aspirated. Continuous aspiration has been associated with acute hypoxemia, arrhythmia, and death. Prophylactic antibiotics are not required during intubation. Endotracheal tubes must be cuffed for effective therapy. There are two approaches toward cuffing the tube: 1) maintain the inflated cuff until the endotracheal tube is removed; and 2) deflate the cuff periodically. Both approaches attempt to reduce the incidence of tracheal stenosis and ulcerations. We know of no systematic approach to the problem but favor deflating the cuff periodically. Before deflating the cuff the naso- and oropharynx should be aspirated of accumulated debris and secretions. Otherwise they will be aspirated into the trachea.

Tracheostomy is much less commonly performed. When it does become necessary, the same care and management must be exercised as for endotracheal tubes. The inner cannula must be removed and cleaned periodically. It appears that the greatest incidence of tracheal stenosis is associated with the Portex plastic tube, and for this reason metal cannulae are now used exclusively. Tracheostomy must be considered after 5 to 6 days of endotracheal intubation. Longer periods of intubation jeopardize the vocal cords as well as the trachea. We have seen endotracheal tubes in place for almost a week without harm, but it is customary to perform tracheostomy after 5 to 6 days.

CONTROL OF METABOLIC ACIDOSIS

Metabolic acidosis rarely amounts to a serious problem in the patient with an uncomplicated myocardial infarction. Metabolic acidosis appears immediately after cardiac arrest and is proportional to the duration of circulatory embarrassment. It must be corrected promptly in order to successfully defibrillate the heart. Correction is made by administering $NaHCO_3$ intravenously. The following formula may be used as a guide.

$$[\text{Buffer base* (normal)} - \text{Buffer base (observed)}] \times \text{ECF}$$
$$or \ [\text{Bicarbonate (normal)} - \text{Bicarbonate (observed)}] \times \text{ECF}$$
$$\text{ECF} = 20\% \text{ of body weight in Kg.}$$

This amount of sodium can usually be administered without fear of precipitating congestive heart failure. A bolus of bicarbonate may be injected initially and subsequent determinations made of the arterial pH. Further bicarbonate therapy should be less vigorous.

Bicarbonate is supplied in vials of 44 mEq per 50 cc or as a 5 percent solution for intravenous administration. During prolonged resuscitation it is more efficient to suspend a bottle of 500 cc of 5 percent sodium bicarbonate and let it run in freely until the patient regains spontaneous circulation. Overcorrection of acidosis is no problem. The patient compensates for this by "blowing off" excess bicarbonate. Excess sodium may be dealt with by prescribing appropriate diuretics such as furosemide or ethacrynic acid.

THE "A, B, C's" OF HEART LUNG RESUSCITATION (SAFAR)

The simplicity of mnemonics has been very effectively used by Dr. Peter Safar for teaching resuscitation.

A—airway—tilt the head back
B—breathe
C—cannulate—closed-chest massage
D—drugs
E—ECG
F—fibrillation treatment
G—gauge—evaluate the cause

---

* Buffer base represents bicarbonate stores. In venous blood CO_2 content includes both HCO_3 and CO_2. According to the Henderson-Hessebach equation, CO_2 is a small fraction of CO_2 content and for practical purposes total CO_2 content = bicarbonate reserve. In arterial blood actual bicarbonate is measured indirectly and expressed as mEq/liter. Either unit may be substituted in the formula.

H—hypothermia if patient remains unconscious

I—intensive care

Dr. Safar's instructions, as above, can be obtained in card form (for wallet) or as a poster (American Heart Association, 44 E. 23rd Street, New York, New York 10010).

Similarly, the letters VIP are used for teaching purposes.

V—ventilate (airway and respirators)

I—infuse (drugs)

P—perfuse (closed-chest massage)

References

Adgey, J., Nelson, P. G., Scott, M. E., Geddes, J. S., Allen, J. D., Zaidi, J. A., and Pantridge, J. F. Management of ventricular fibrillation outside hospital. Lancet, 1:1169, 1969.

Fletcher, G. F. Hazardous complication of closed chest cardiac massage. Amer. Heart J., 77:431, 1969.

Grace, W. J., and Minogue, W. F. Resuscitation for cardiac arrest due to myocardial infarction. Dis. Chest, 50:173, 1966.

Gregory, J. J., and Grace, W. J. Resuscitation of the severely ill patient with acute myocardial infarction. Amer. J. Cardiol., 20: 836, 1967.

Jude, J. R., and Elam, J. O. Fundamentals of Cardiopulmonary Resuscitation. Philadelphia, F. A. Davis Co., 1965.

Kouwenhoven, W. B., Jude, J. R., and Knickerbocker, G. G. Closed chest cardiac massage. J.A.M.A., 173:1064, 1960.

Morgan, R., and Grace, W. J. Laceration of the liver from closed chest cardiac massage. New Eng. J. Med., 265:82, 1961.

Minogue, W. F., Smessart, A. A., and Grace, W. J. External cardiac massage for cardiac arrest due to myocardial infarction. A changing concept. Amer. J. Cardiol., 13:25, 1964.

Nachlas, N. M., and Miller, D. I. Closed chest cardiac resuscitation in patients with acute myocardial infarction. Amer. Heart J., 69:448, 1965.

Phillips, J. H., and Burch, H. E. Management of cardiac arrest. Amer. Heart J., 67:265, 1964.

Robinson, J. S., Sloman, G., and Mathew, T. H. Survival after resuscitation from cardiac arrest in acute myocardial infarction. Amer. Heart J., 69:740, 1965.

Safar, P. Mouth to airway emergency artificial respiration. J.A.M.A., 196:1459, 1958.

9

Nursing Aspects of
The Coronary Care Unit

The Nurse

Throughout this volume much attention has been paid to the natural history of patients with acute myocardial infarction and to the mechanical aspects of the cardiac monitoring (the hardware). Now we must consider the nurse, the backbone of the Coronary Care Unit without whose knowledge and skill the Unit is destined to fail. Too much emphasis cannot be placed on the importance of her role (software of the Coronary Care Unit).

Over many years considerable social forces have been at work attempting to remove the nurse from the bedside of the patient. Years ago it was felt beneath the diginity of a lady to work as a nurse at the bedside. In recent years it has been felt that the role of the nurse is not at the bedside, but at the administrator's desk. The Coronary Care Unit, as well as the Intensive Care Unit, moves the nurse back to the bedside of the patient. Some feel that the presence of the cardiac monitor and the defibrillator is a further encroachment on the nurse's time. Actually, monitors assist the nurses in rendering better care by making possible more precise observations of the vital signs including the electrocardiographic rhythm. We must emphasize the fact that skillful bedside nurses are not plentiful, and we can no longer afford the luxury of wasting the valuable skills of those available on tasks that can be better assigned to persons of lesser educational background. In this stage of the growth of medicine when the technical aspects of managing the very ill patient are increasing and there is a particularly increased demand for nursing skills, it is of paramount importance that the nurse be relieved of all or many of the multitude of non-nursing responsibilities.

The nurses, especially the charge nurse, should be relieved of some, if not all, of the following:

1. Admission and discharge of patients.
2. Preparation and distribution of patient's food and drink.
3. Stripping and making unoccupied beds.
4. Light housekeeping, such as dusting and locker cleaning, and checking such equipment.
5. Receiving and making telephone calls.
6. Tasks related to the general administration of the ward such as:
   a) Making out time schedules for other nurses.
   b) Clinical duty such as putting lab reports in the charts.
   c) Ordering supplies.

In hospitals without a house staff, or where there is no full time physician in charge of the Intensive Care or Coronary Care Unit, the nurse will be called upon to make increasingly important decisions. In order that she be prepared to do this, special educational programs must be started and continuous educational programs provided.

Nursing Personnel

It should be planned on each shift to have one nurse on duty who is adept at reading the monitor, who is informed about the complications of acute heart disease, and who has been properly instructed and is experienced in a program of cardiac resuscitation. Such a nurse will have been instructed in cardiac monitoring, resuscitation, mouth-to-mouth respiration, and electrical defibrillation. How many cardiac patients such a nurse can take care of is related to her own skills and the assistance she has. Certainly she can take care of more than three patients, but probably less than six. The number of nursing aides and other types of help on the Coronary Care Unit will determine the number of patients with whom a single graduate nurse can deal. In smaller community hosiptals more responsibility will be delegated to the nurse than in larger teaching hospitals which have a house staff.

Hospitals Without House Staffs

In institutions without house staffs, or where there are no physicians on duty full time, the graduate nurse in charge of the unit must have immediate access via telephone to the supervising physician. It is not practical for one physician to answer the telephone seven days a week. Many institutions have adopted a committee of physicians who will be on call at the other end of a "hot line telephone" to the nurse at any time of the day, every day of the week. Such systems have been effective and useful.

In institutions where there is a house staff available, one house officer is generally designated as the responsible person with whom the nurse may be in immediate contact. In hospitals with larger house staffs, an intern or resident may be assigned to the Coronary Care Unit on permanent assignment. In our own institution, where the Coronary Care and Intensive Care Units are adjacent, we assign one first year resident to this double responsibility. This resident may not leave the floor at any time unless he is relieved by a physician of equal competence. It is his responsibility to keep the nurse abreast of continuing changes in the patient's medical condition and whenever possible to teach the nurse so that she may render better patient care.

Nurses Responsibilities in the Monitoring Unit

Nurses who have been specially instructed in cardiology and in the technique of cardiac resuscitation and who are assigned either to the Emergency Room or the Cardiac Monitoring Unit should be delegated authority by the hospital to perform the following procedures:

1. Attach electrodes to the patient and maintain constant ECG monitoring.
2. Take an electrocardiogram.
3. Perform any part of closed chest cardiac resuscitation (see joint statements of AMA, CNA, January 1965).
4. Perform electric defibrillation.
5. Start and maintain inhalation therapy (i.e., assisted ventilation, using respirators) when the inhalation therapy personnel are not immediately available.
6. Initiate rotating tourniquets on patients with acute heart failure and acute pulmonary edema.

In some hospitals, where circumstances demand it:

7. *The nurse may insert intravenous medication directly into the tubing of an intravenous catheter in an undiluted state on the physician's orders.* The following drugs are examples: Heparin, sodium bicarbonate, digoxin, corticosteroid, xylocaine, Pronestyl, antibiotics.
8. The nurse, after suitable training, may start an intravenous setup of dextrose in water.

MENTAL ALARMS VERSUS ELECTRONIC ALARMS

Part of education of the career nurse in charge of the Coronary Care Unit must be a knowledge of the natural course of the patient with acute myocardial infarction. Depending on the nurses involved, more or less responsibility can be delegated. Institutions will vary and each must make its own protocol. There are certain circumstances, however, when immediate action must be the response to certain symptoms; for example, the patient in the Coronary Care Unit who: 1) suddenly loses consciousness; 2) has a general convulsion; 3) suddenly begins to perspire and has a weak or feeble pulse. Such events clearly indicate a drastic change in the cardiac output and an imminent catastrophe.

Here the nurse must take the following action with what help is available:

1. Notifies the physician (electric code system is preferable).
2. Provides the respirator and starts it, after checking the airway.
3. Provides the defibrillator, plugs it in, and prepares the paddles.
4. Provides an I.V. set if one is not running and starts it if a physician is not available.
5. Provides the crash cart.

6. Obtains an ECG rhythm strip. If the patient becomes pulseless at any point during this time, the nurse should defibrillate him immediately. If the patient is having ventricular tachycardia with failing blood pressure, or rapid atrial fibrillation with falling blood pressure, the nurse should defibrillate the patient immediately.

The above sequence in our institution constitutes an emergency calling for a "code." On pushing a button in the wall, a signal is activated in the telephone room (Chap. 2, Fig. 5). The telephone room personnel then announce over the loudspeaker, "*Code 99,*" which is our signal for an all-out resuscitation effort.

There are other less critical circumstances that call for prompt attention which cannot be delegated or abrogated until the crises subside. *Here the nurse must mobilize for action.* For example, when:
1. the patient becomes short of breath;
2. the pulse rate increases by more than 25 beats/minute for more than 60 seconds;
3. the heart rate falls below 50;
4. A/V dissociation develops;
5. VPC's appear at the rate of one per 6 seconds (one per sweep of oscilloscope);
6. VPC's occur in groups of two or more;
7. there is a marked change in cardiac rhythm; sinus rhythm to atrial fibrillation with a rapid ventricular rate.

When any of the above occur, the nurse will:
1. run a strip of electrocardiogram;
2. attach all leads for performing a 12-lead electrocardiogram;
3. call for the physician;
4. inspect the patient's airway to see if it is adequate and patent;
5. bring up and plug in the defibrillator;
6. record the blood pressure every minute for 4 or 5 minutes;
7. if there is no I.V. running bring the necessary equipment to the bedside with the equipment for a cutdown and for the insertion of a central venous catheter;
8. in the event of onset of multiple VPC's, notify the physician, bring up the I.V. equipment, and draw up the Xylocaine, 50 mg, in a syringe.

Other changes in vital signs call for alertness, but of lesser degree than the above: *Here the nurse must monitor the patient very closely.*
1. Change in heart rate of 20/min.

2. Persistent chest pain.
3. Sudden change in ECG rhythm.

The nurse should run frequent ECG rhythm strips, start oxygen, record vital signs every 15 minutes, and notify the physician in charge.

WRITING ORDERS IN ADVANCE

In some institutions where no full-time physicians are on the unit and no physician is predictably in the hospital, orders are written in advance. For example, the order is written that if "the patient's electrocardiogram shows more than one VPC per 6 seconds the patient is to be given intravenous Lidocaine immediately." Any variety of medication or circumstances can be conceived under the above scheme and written on the nurse's order sheet. This, then, puts considerable responsibility on the charge nurse for decision-making but does relieve her of some of the legal responsibility. If one is going to adopt this contingent ordering, it is imperative that all in the hospital, including the Board of Trustees, be aware of and agree to what is being done.

Standing Orders:
Patients with Acute
or Suspect of Acute
Myocardial Infarction

Patients are admitted to a Coronary Care Unit from a wide area: the ambulance on call, the attending physician at the patient's home or his office, the resident physician in the Emergency Room, or a physician in the community. The patient often arrives on the Coronary Care Unit without specific instruction, and it is left to the nurse to decide what to do in the interim. The first few hours in the hospital are the most critical for the patient. In the absence of specific instructions, standing orders should be adopted by the nursing staff, after consultation with the medical staff. The following are typical of such orders:

ELECTROCARDIOGRAM

An electrocardiogram must be taken on every patient who is not admitted directly from the clinic or the emergency room, or who does not bring an electrocardiogram with him. Repeat the ECG if it is more than four hours old. The nurses will automatically order an electrocardiogram, to be done "stat," if one is not immediately available. Patients with acute myocardial infarction should have daily electrocardiograms for the first four hospital days.

VITAL SIGNS

Blood pressure, pulse, and respiration rates are recorded every hour for the first 2 hours, then every 4 hours. Temperature is taken orally every 4 hours.

OXYGEN

All patients with recent myocardial infarction will receive oxygen at 6 liters per minute by nasal cannula.

FLUIDS

Intake and output of fluids will be recorded. An intravenous setup of dextrose and water with a micro drip will be started and maintained to keep the vein patent in all "coronary patients."

ELECTRODES

The electrodes will be immediately attached to the patient by the nurse when notified of the diagnosis of acute myocardial infarct. The needles should be inserted subcutaneously on the chest wall to approximate the lead from the standard electrocardiogram with the tallest R wave (see page 31). Care should be taken not to insert a needle electrode into breast tissue in the female. This can be avoided by placing the needle laterally on the chest wall. The anterior surface of the chest wall should be kept free of tape and needles in case defibrillation or cardioversion is necessary. The electrodes must be changed by the nurse every 2 or 3 days or more frequently if necessary. Excessive electrical interference or diminishing R wave amplitude usually indicates that new electrodes are necessary.

MONITORING OF THE PATIENT WHILE CHANGING THE BED OR WHILE GIVING A BATH

While the patient's bed is being changed, or while he is being given a bed bath, electric currents from muscle contraction are produced which activate the high frequency alarm. In order to avoid this, the nurse is permitted to set the high frequency alarm indicator at 250 for such periods of nursing care. The alarms are *not* to be turned off during these times, as this would also block out the "low frequency" alarm which must be kept active. The alarms may be turned off only if the needles are to be removed from the chest or replaced, which happens every 48 hours.

RESTRICTIONS

No smoking is permitted. No bedside radios are permitted except those with an earpiece. No phone calls are permitted.

DIET

Until otherwise changed, the following diet will be given: 1,600 calorie, low cholesterol, low fat diet. The patient should be encouraged to eat but never forced. Many patients experience anorexia in the first few days of myocardial infarction. Patients may be helped with their meals, depending upon how much distress they appear to have. There is no real reason why they should be spoon-fed, but someone should stand by to see that they do not overstretch or overtax themselves physically.

BED REST

All patients with transmural myocardial infarction, or suspected of the same, shall be placed on complete bed rest until this order is changed. The usual duration of rest is 2 to 4 days. The physician may be reminded to change it any time after the fourth day. The patient may assume a reclining position on either side and may be permitted to sit up at a 45 degree angle from time to time, but he is not permitted to dangle his feet over the side of the bed or to stand unaided. If the patient is having exceptional difficulty emptying his bladder while lying in bed, he may be permitted to stand up in order to do so, provided the orderly is standing beside him. This position may not be assumed without the physician's written permission. With written permission, the patient may use a bedside commode or may be assisted to the bathroom for a bowel movement at any time. Otherwise, patients are encouraged to use a commode at the bedside.

BEDPAN; BEDSIDE COMMODE; BATHROOM PRIVILEGES

There is little or no scientific evidence that a patient with a recent acute myocardial infarction is better treated if he uses the bed pan in the bed for bowel movements than if he is allowed to take a few steps to the bathroom. Traditionally, the hospitalized patient with acute myocardial infarction is ordered to "complete bed rest" which, in our institution, means that he must use the bed pan. Patients are allowed to use the bedside commode after the first hospital day. Whether or not the patient may be allowed to go to a bathroom depends more upon the availability of such a facility and an attendant to accompany him, than on the established harm or good that may come of such activity. More and more, bedside commodes are being used. Recently, a portable septic tank (reusable flush toilet) has been acquired, and it is probable that such a device will be widely accepted (see Chap. 3, Fig. 1). Its use will probably settle this problem for some time to come.

The patient should be shaved by the attendant daily. For patients who are not critically ill, the usual partial bed bath may be given by the ward attendant.

Except for patients who are critically ill, passive exercises of the legs and feet are to be encouraged at all times.

ENZYME STUDIES

All patients suspected of having acute myocardial infarction will have a determination of LDH, SGOT, and CPK ordered daily for 3 days. The order is discontinued if the first "set" is grossly abnormal.

VISITORS

No more than two visitors at any one time for no more than 5 minutes per hour.

CRITICAL PATIENTS

All patients being monitored for acute myocardial infarction are "on critical." All patients in shock and heart failure are "on critical." Some patients with arrhythmias should be "on critical."

DURATION OF CARDIAC MONITORING

Patients with acute myocardial infarction should be monitored for 7 to 10 days if they have a transmural myocardial infarction. Patients with "rule out" myocardial infarction, and those who have "non-transmural myocardial infarction," should be monitored for 3 days or less. From analysis of our own data, it is becoming increasingly clear that the frightful accident of sudden unexpected ventricular fibrillation may occur at almost any time during the first 14 hospital days.

DISCHARGE FROM THE CARDIAC MONITORING UNIT

Once the period of monitoring is over, the patient will be discharged from the CCU on order of the house staff, the personal physician of the patient, or the director of the unit. Any conflict as to priority for discharge will be settled by the Director of Medicine. No private patient will be discharged without previous communication with the personal attending physician.

Routine transfer out of the CCU should occur during the daytime and not after 8 P.M. After that time, if there are no beds in the CCU, the patients who are admitted to the hospital with the diagnosis of acute myocardial infarction can be held in the Emergency Room where there is a cardiac monitor until a CCU bed becomes available. It is prudent to keep one bed empty at night to provide a safety valve for emergency night admissions. Patients should not be moved out of the CCU after 8 P.M. in order to make room for others. Actually, the largest impediment to discharge of the patient from the Coronary Care Unit has been the lack of available beds in the general hospital. Since instituting an Intermediate Coronary Care Unit, the problem has been less troublesome due to better all-around communication and the availability of a special place to transfer the patients.

An occasional physician will wish to have his patient remain in the Coronary Care Unit, but without the ECG monitor. This is not acceptable and such a patient must be moved off the unit. If a patient is not being monitored in the CCU, a bed is being wasted.

ROUTINE ORDERS AND POLICIES DURING EMERGENCY

Certain routine orders in regard to patients with acute myocardial infarction are contained in above sections. Although all physicians are expected to be familiar with the techniques of cardiopulmonary resuscitation and emergency defibrillation, it is not practical to consider that all attending physicians wish to participate in these procedures, or consider themselves expert. With this in mind, it is our policy during emergency procedures to have the ranking medical resident in charge of the emergency procedure. In the event of the presence of the attending physician, he may delegate this responsibility to the resident, or take charge himself.

The preceding set of orders is suggested as a guideline and is by no means intended to be rigid or complete. The variety and detail of standing orders are related to the availability of a physician's constant attendance on the Coronary Unit. Standing orders are not intended to be a substitute for thinking and should be altered to suit a particular clinical situation.

SEDATION

Almost all patients are given sedation at night. Certain patients may require sedation, in which event phenobarbital is given. Phenothiazines are not given to these patients because shock may develop, which phenothiazine may aggravate. No routine daytime sedation is given or is needed.

A Suggested System of Patient Priorities in the CCU

ADMISSION AND TRANSFER OF PATIENTS TO THE CARDIAC MONITORING UNIT

Patients are referred to the CCU by private attending physicians, by physicians working in the Out-Patient Department, and by resident physicians in the Emergency Room or the Out-Patient Department. The physicians may refer their patients directly to the CCU. In the event that they decide that the patient has an acute myocardial infarction, or is suspected of having such, their opinion is never seriously challenged by the physicians in charge of the Coronary Care Unit. We feel it is preferable to accept the patient and to be sure of the diagnosis, even though a few days may be spent doing this. There is always the possibility that the initial ECG and physical examination will be within normal limits, even though the patient may ultimately show the changes of acute myocardial infarction. Inasmuch as the majority of the deaths occur on day one or day two, it is better to be safe than sorry.

In referring the patient to the Cardiac Monitoring Unit the physicians and nurses must separate the patients into three groups so that they may be subgrouped together if the unit is large, or separated from one another if the circumstances demand different types of nursing care. We use the following schema as a guide:

GROUP I: Patients with acute myocardial infarction, uncomplicated.

GROUP II: Arrhythmia problems and problems necessitating electric pacemakers without acute myocardial infarction (cardiac monitoring).

GROUP III: Patients in shock, or acute pulmonary edema with acute myocardial infarction.

GROUP I

A. The patient with uncomplicated acute myocardial infarction.
B. The patient with non-transmural infarction.
C. The patient suspected of having acute myocardial infarction.

It is felt that the life of the Group I patient depends upon constant attention to the electrocardiographic monitor for the early detection and prompt treatment of life-threatening arrhythmias. If the monitor is not scrutinized almost continuously, we are not protecting the patient and cannot say we are doing cardiac monitoring.

The patients in Group I should be placed together if the Coronary Care Unit has several beds per room. These patients should be separate from those with acute myocardial infarction who need intensive nursing care (Group III), and from those whose needs for nursing care are less demanding (Group II, arrhythmia without A.M.I.). This separation may not be clear-cut and frequent compromises are required, often resulting in Group I and II patients being adjacent to one another. Patients in Group III are always moved into an Intensive Care Unit and clearly separated from patients in Group I and II.

DURATION OF MONITORING—GROUP I

A) The patients with acute transmural myocardial infarction are monitored for 7 to 10 days and for at least 5 days after the last arrhythmia. Once again our major responsibility here is meticulous attention to the monitors. Any deviation from standards established for heart rate (50-120), or change in rhythm, must be reported immediately. It is generally felt that by the time 7 to 10 days have elapsed 90 percent of the accidents in this type of patient will have occurred and that the patient may be transferred with considerable security. Our current practice is to transfer such a patient to an Intermediate Coronary Care Unit, which we describe in another section.

B) The patient with non-transmural infarction (subendocardial infarction; intramural infarction) is to be monitored for 48 hours only, provided he becomes asymptomatic immediately. Or, preferably, he is monitored for 48 hours after becoming asymptomatic. He is then transferred to the I.C.C.U.

C) Patients who are suspected of having acute myocardial infarction: We feel that the diagnosis of transmural or non-transmural infarction should become clear after 48 hours of observation. If, at this time, the ECG remains stable and no enzyme changes have taken place, the patient may then be discharged from the hospital or transferred to the general hospital.

We have an occasional practitioner who refers his patient to the Cardiac Monitoring Unit but does not wish his patient to be on the monitor. We do not accept this situation. Unless the patient is on the monitor we cannot keep him on the unit, as someone else will need this bed and monitor.

Patients in Group I have absolute priority for monitored beds. In the event that there are more patients and/or beds than there are monitors, monitors may be removed from the patients in the other categories in order to give them to Group I patients.

GROUP II (CARDIAC ARRHYTHMIA MONITORING)

This group consists of patients without myocardial infarction who are being monitored because they are subject to paroxysmal tachycardia, electric pacemaker problems, or other kinds of arrhythmias. Generally, such patients do not require such careful and meticulous monitor attention, and it is quite satisfactory to set the alarm rates at predetermined levels and to pay attention to the monitor only when the alarm rings. Needless to say, the alarm should be turned on. These patients are monitored only as long as they are in a state of crisis. Some are monitored for only a few hours, then cardioverted, and discharged from CCU. Others, such as patients with arrhythmia due to digitalis toxicity, may be monitored for a few days.

It might be questioned why such a patient is kept on the so-called Coronary Care Unit. The technical skill involved in continuous electrocardiographic monitoring and the know-how of the nursing staff in taking care of such patients with cardiac arrhythmia is not general and is not supplied throughout the hospital. Since it is available in only one area, such patients are monitored in the CCU.

GROUP III

These are patients who have an acute myocardial infarction with catastrophic-type complications, namely shock or acute pulmonary edema. These patients are no longer placed in the Coronary Monitoring Unit or in the Cardiac Monitoring Area. In our hospital they are placed in an adjacent station which we refer to as the "shock room." In other institutions they are placed in Intensive Care Units. In general, it is felt that such patients who are desperately sick are better away from those patients with uncomplicated myocardial infarction because of the possible emotional effect that desperate illness produces in others.

Monitoring for such patients is necessary, but their lives really depend on other methods designed to treat shock and acute pulmonary edema, and not essentially on electrocardiographic monitoring. The intensive nursing and medical care which they receive will more probably determine the outcome than the nature of the cardiac arrhythmias. Consequently, such patients probably do not need continuous electrocardiographic monitoring if there is another patient who needs it more because of serious arrhythmia.

EMPTY BEDS

Cardiac monitoring beds are quite precious and must be utilized. One should be kept open awaiting a patient, even if other types of patients need hospitalization. This is quite contrary to general hospital administration practices, where all the beds must be occupied. On the other hand, it is the responsibility of the unit to determine its own bed needs and to keep these beds filled. It destroys the entire concept and is bad for all of the patients if patients with non-coronary and non-arrhythmia problems are admitted to such a Cardiac Monitoring Unit.

The priority system for beds is of the same order as the priority system for the monitors. Patients from Group II can be moved out of the unit to make room for patients in Group I. These priority decisions must always be made in advance and all of the physicians in the hospital must be made aware of this practice so that there will be no undue discussion at the time concerning any individual patient. The Coronary Care Unit exists for the Group I patients. The unit also serves patients in Groups II and III but never at the expense of the patients in Group I.

The Technician's Role in the Coronary Care Unit

THE PARAMEDICAL PERSONNEL

Much is being required of the physician and nurse today, far beyond and different from the classic conception of physicians' skills or intensive nursing care. This includes knowledge of electronic monitors, respirators, defibrillators, and techniques such as closed-chest resuscitation. There is no reason to feel that the nurses must continue to learn and relearn the use of every new mechanical or electrical instrument that comes into being; we will be wasting precious nursing skills. Such instruments, devices, and techniques can be taught to highly motivated young people who have not had the extensive education of nurses. Technicians can be hired out of a pool of people which is not as yet being exhausted. These people should work under the direction of the physician in charge of the unit. Such people as operators of ECG machines, monitoring devices, and respirator devices could be taught to relieve the nurse of many technical responsibilities, thus freeing nurses' time for more meticulous attention to physical signs, bedside observation, and application of clinical skills (not for more administrative work).

THE USE OF PARAMEDICAL PERSONNEL IN THE CORONARY CARE UNIT

The essence of lowering mortality rates in patients with an acute myocardial infarction is meticulous and constant observation of the electrocardiographic monitoring bank. Unless the patient is having constant electrocardiographic monitoring, early warning signs of impending disaster may be overlooked and significant opportunities for introducing life-saving therapy to abort life-threatening arrhythmias will be missed. Considerable experience has indicated that although resuscitation from life-threatening arrhythmia, such as ventricular fibrillation, is practical and workable, the opportunity to avoid the necessity for resuscitation is of uppermost importance.

When we instituted the Coronary Care Unit at St. Vincent's Hospital in 1963, the system consisted of simply setting the alarm rates at high and low frequency limits and waiting for the alarm to ring. In time we realized that this was not the most appropriate way to proceed, and it was decided that a physician should sit in front of the ECG monitor bank and observe the ECG monitors regularly, 24 hours per day, every day of the week. This proved to be impractical from a logistic point of view and had to be abandoned. It was therefore decided that graduate nurses specially trained in cardiology and electrocardiography should sit in front of the monitor bank on a 24-hour basis to detect early warning signs of impending disaster. This, too, proved to be impractical from the same point of view because 1) very few nurses were available; 2) nurses in general do not like to sit in front of such an arrangement without any significant break in the routine day after day, or even hour after hour, except to leave the monitors in order to attend a patient who is in trouble; and 3) increasing awareness that this is not proper duty for nurses. Consequently, although we had the monitors observed regularly (at least on paper) by the nursing staff, this did not prove useful or practical.

It was then decided that electrocardiographic technicians could be taught the fundamentals of cardiology. They could work as suitable substitutes for nurses and physicians. Since February 1, 1968, we have used electrocardiographic technicians trained by us to observe the monitor bank on a 24-hour basis. Time and experience have proven that this is a useful and practical device. These young people have quickly learned the rudiments of electrocardiographic interpretation of the arrhythmias and how to evaluate and separate serious arrhythmias from false alarms and other artefacts on the oscilloscopes. They make a rhythm strip hourly, mount these in order, and present them to the person in charge, hourly (Fig. 1).

More than one clear-cut example is available to indicate that an alert electrocardiographic technician has detected ventricular fibrillation and after documenting this has promptly notified the nurse with the result that the patient was defibrillated within 30 seconds of the

ST. VINCENT'S HOSPITAL
AND MEDICAL CENTER OF NEW YORK

HISTORY and PROGRESS NOTES

DATE   *9-23-69*

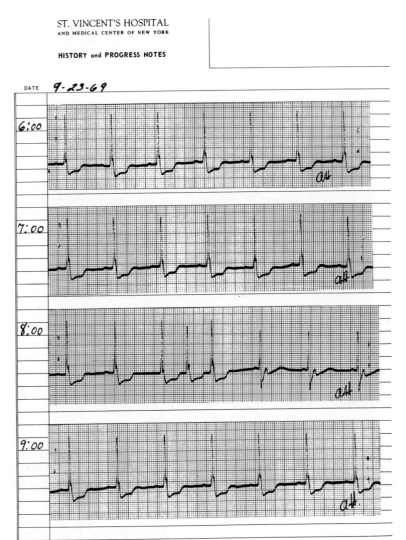

Fig. 1. Rhythm strips are recorded hourly and mounted to become a permanent record. The strips are reviewed promptly by a member of the house staff and initialed. Any change in cardiac rhythm is recorded by the monitor bank technician and brought immediately to the attention of a physician.

onset of the arrhythmia. This practice makes available another supply of manpower, not previously utilized, and may stimulate young people to enter new fields (nursing).

The second category of paramedical personnel we are using in the Coronary Care Unit is the highly skilled electronic technician. He is assigned a small space in which to work in the area of the Intensive Care Unit, and his responsibility is to service all electronic apparatus, including the electrocardiograph machines of the hospital (Chap. 2, Fig. 12). This man has proven to be very useful. He makes repairs immediately so that in the past year no electronic equipment has been sent out of the hospital for repairs and no apparatus has been out of service for more than 48 hours. In addition, this technician acts as a handyman consulting with the nurses to solve their problems with the electrical apparatus and other kinds of mechanical devices used on the Intensive Care Unit and the Coronary Care Unit. Such mechanical and electronic knowledge is a great help to nursing staff in the use, repair, and maintenance of equipment.

In the course of time we have embarked on the training of the electronic technicians, as well as electronic repairmen, to participate in resuscitation procedures and the use of the electric defibrillator for cardioversion. This is rehearsed on a weekly training basis to the point where the electronic technician can participate with the house staff in elective cardioversion and emergency defibrillation without the house staff or the nurses having to be responsible for any part of the electrical apparatus. In these days of increasing shortage of nurses and increasing utilization of more and more complicated electrical equipment, it is unlikely that we will be able to find the number of nurses we need and it is unreasonable that we insist upon their acting as electrical engineers. Consequently, the employment of skilled electronic technicians on the unit is useful and, in our experience, quite workable.

Teaching Cardiac Resuscitation

A system of continuing education must be established for the staff. This responsibility usually rests with the Director of Medicine but may be shared by the head nurse in the Coronary Care Unit if she herself has participated in an accredited educational program.

Because of the urgency of cardiac arrest, it is imperative that all individuals working with the patients be expert in the techniques of resuscitation, whether they are interns, residents, attending physicians, or nurses. It is frequently stated that the patient may survive cardiac arrest for as long as 3 to 4 minutes without circulation. Although this may be applicable to 18-year-olds, it is certainly far from accurate in those who are in the coronary artery disease age group and who have had an acute myocardial infarction. It is likely that in such patients the situation becomes irreversible after less than 60 seconds without circulation. Therefore, almost no harm can be done by anyone who attempts to restore the circulation in a patient with cardiac arrest.

Each nurse who works on the Coronary Care Unit and in the Intensive Care Unit is instructed in the technique of closed-chest cardiac massage, and supervised during actual attempts at resuscitation. The technique of electrical defibrillation is taught to the nurses in the Animal Experimental Laboratory, using the anesthetized dog (Fig. 2). Classes are held every week for approximately one and one-half hours, and every nurse who works on this service is taught to handle

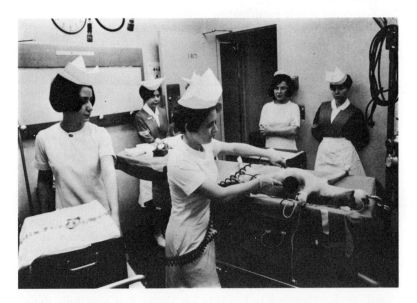

Fig. 2. A method of instructing nurses in the technique of defibrillation. An anesthetized dog is connected to a cardiac monitor. The dog is not sacrificed and suffers no ill effect. Suitable booby traps are introduced and the nurse is timed to her best effort.

the electrical defibrillation equipment and must do so repeatedly until it is felt she is capable of doing this alone. We then inform the hospital staff that the nurse on duty may carry out electrical defibrillation of the heart within 30 seconds of the detection of this event, if a physician has not arrived within this time. It is a rewarding experience to see how quickly the nurses master the procedure and how efficient they become. It is likely that they can learn to handle the equipment better than the physicians as they participate in all of the cardiac resuscitations whereas any one physician participates only in a few cases.

HANDLING OF THE DEFIBRILLATION EQUIPMENT

Personnel using the equipment must be rehearsed in a rigid systematic manner so that no one will be accidentally injured or burned. Common errors in handling the equipment are:
1. Holding both paddles in one hand when the apparatus is "charged."
2. Too many people participating so that:
    a. the "button" may be pushed at the wrong time;
    b. both paddles are left on top of the instrument when the instrument is being "charged";
    c. too much electrode jelly is placed on the patient's skin so that the current may flow from one paddle to the other without flowing through the heart;
    d. people at the bedside have their hands in contact with the patient at the time the current is delivered;
    e. there is failure to have good skin contact with the whole surface of the paddle.

Only one code word should be used to activate the equipment, e.g., "hit it!" During the excitement of a resuscitation attempt, many people will be saying "O.K.", "Go ahead", "I'm ready", and unless a standard code word is used someone may push the button at the wrong time.

The team of physicians and nurses must be repeatedly rehearsed, preferably using the Animal Laboratory or some suitable simulator. Considerable experience in this field has shown that any "little thing" will delay the defibrillation procedure, e.g., the physician using new equipment may need 3 to 4 minutes before he is ready; the nurse, unable to locate the electrode jelly, delays the procedure; the drawer of the table, being overloaded with unnecessary equipment, may delay the procedure 1 to 2 minutes. The usual patient with ventricular fibrillation does not have 3 to 4 minutes to live without circulation—he probably has 60 seconds or less.

Although one can provide some circulation with closed-chest massage, the cardiac output provided by the defibrillated heart is much more effective. In order for nurses to become skillful, a good deal of education and practical experience is necessary. The following educational technique has been worked out in this institution and has been in practice weekly for over three years. Nurses are permitted to do emergency defibrillation in the Coronary Care Unit after this training period. This procedure has been approved by the executive committee of the hospital.

A TEACHING METHOD

A mongrel dog is lightly anesthetized with pentobarbital, an endotracheal tube is inserted, and a respirator is placed on standby. The dog is monitored by a commercial electrocardiographic monitoring system. The electric defibrillator is brought into the room and the instrument is thoroughly explained to the nurses. The nurses then progress stepwise through the procedure of activating the instrument, applying electrode jelly to the paddles, applying the paddles to the dog, and delivering the electric current; the apparatus is then deactivated. The femoral pulse of the dog is palpated before and after the "defibrillation." The exercise is limited to three to five nurses at one time.

Emphasis is placed on avoiding dangerous moves, such as holding two paddles in one hand, waving one paddle in the air, or being in contact with the dog or the table. After two or three trials in one morning, the nurses are then encouraged to move more quickly; and the final exercise of the morning consists of timing the nurses, using a stopwatch, from the word, "Go," until the dog is "defibrillated." At this first session, generally, no further work is done except to check out the speed and the nurses' knowledge of the equipment. On subsequent days, the apparatus is "bugged" and booby traps are introduced into the room to delay the nurse, or to distract her from functioning properly, unless she is thoroughly familiar with the machine. Under these circumstances, the nurses are timed with the stopwatch.

The following chart shows some of the causes of delays in defibrillation:

TIME REQUIRED TO DEFIBRILLATE

30 seconds	Shortest possible time
65 seconds	Could not get the cap off the jelly tube
90 seconds	Could not find the electrical socket
2 minutes +	No jelly on the cart
65 seconds	Pushed wrong switch
75 seconds	Too many wires in the drawer

After the nurses have attended three successive sessions, usually at weekly intervals, they are not required to return for a period of a month or longer. They are then tested again to see how proficient they are, and the above procedures are generally repeated.

At the beginning of these sessions attempts were made to produce ventricular fibrillation in the animal, using alternating current and/or intravenous digitalis. These maneuvers proved too lethal for the animals and did not contribute to the training process.

COMMENT

This course is well received by the Nursing Service and the morale of the group doing the procedures is high. The cost should be minimal. The same dog is used over and over again, apparently with no particular harm to the animal. Inasmuch as the animal is sedated, he seems to have no memory of the event and greets the anesthetist happily each morning. There has been no risk to the students during this 3-year period. Although a mild shock was received on one occasion, no serious accidents have occurred. In addition, it is of interest to note that the machine was broken and had to be sent to the factory for repairs only once during all of these sessions. At the present time, we are extending this experience to all student nurses of the graduating class. (Our student nurses spend five weeks on the Intensive Care Unit and, during this period of time, each one is given individual instruction on the use of the defibrillator.)

The results of this training are hard to evaluate, except in terms of the survival of patients. In the last 12 months our nurses have defibrillated six patients on their own, with four survivors. It is also quite obvious that the nurses handle the equipment more effectively and more confidently than many house officers.

Recently, simulators have been introduced for pulmonary venti-lation (Recus-Anne) and for defibrillation. The authors strongly encourage such teaching aids.

Education and Orientation of the Patient

When the patient is admitted to the hospital Coronary Care Unit, the nurse describes to the patient the environmental situation. She will tell him what the monitors are being used for, what elec-trodes are for, and how he must handle himself in regard to the wires that are attached to him. She does this in addition to the routine introduction of any patient to the hospital, and explains to him that the wires are connected to electrocardiographic monitors and that these monitors are continuously scrutinized by professional people. This is emphasized to increase the patient's security. The nurse then exam-ines the patient, records his blood pressure, listens to his lungs and heart, and palpates the peripheral pulses as a point of future refer-ence. During her daily inspection the nurse repeats the above type of physical examination and encourages the patient each day that he is making further progress towards discharge from the Coronary Care Unit to the Intermediate Coronary Care System. She is free to point out that the bulk of patients admitted to the Coronary Care Unit are discharged in good condition. When the patient is ready for discharge the nurse explains to him the Intermediate Coronary Care System. She is free to tell the patient that, by this time, the chances of his going home from the hospital are exceptionally good.

Nurses and physicians should be more aware of the phenomenon called "coronary blues." This catastrophic illness precipitates in many middle-aged people a striking reactive depression. Practically all of the patients experience this, some more than others. It lasts from a few days to a few months, although most of the patients recover before they leave the hospital. It is well to anticipate a mild depres-sion so that the patient will not be thought to have some additional illness accounting for his fatigue and lack of vitality, and will not be thought to be somewhat insane if he seems to be on the verge of tears. The nurse should explain to the patient the "coronary blues" phenomenón. She may help to relieve his anxiety about this experi-ence by explaining its prevalence and stating that it will go away without medication or further hospitalization.

References

Criteria and Guidelines for Nurse Training Courses in Coronary Care Units. U.S. Department of Health, Education, and Welfare.

Grace, W. J. A note on the Teaching of Electrical Defibrillation. Amer. J. Nurs., 70:97, 1970.

Grace, W. J. The use of paramedical personnel in the Coronary Care Unit. Clin. Res., XVII:616, December, 1969.

Nursing in Coronary Care Units. Selected publications, films, and other teaching aids. U.S. Department of Health, Education, and Welfare. Public Health Service Publication 1629, Bibliography No. 74.

Training technics for the coronary care unit. Second Bethesda Conference of the American College of Cardiology. December 11, 12, 1965, Washington, D.C. Amer. J. Cardiol., 17:736, 1966.

10

Intermediate
Coronary Care Unit

Where Does the Patient Go Following Discharge From the CCU?

Referring to Figure 2, Chapter 1 (p. 3), it may be noted that in this series of patients, 30 percent of the deaths that occurred from acute myocardial infarction occurred after leaving the Coronary Care Unit. Approximately half of these deaths were sudden and unexpected. The other half occurred in patients who experienced a complication during the initial phase of their illness, with unstable blood pressure, recurrent arrhythmia, or congestive heart failure. Similar data have been published by others (Oliver et al.). Because half of the deaths were due to the same mechanism as the original threat to life, namely arrhythmia, systems for caring for patients after discharge from the Coronary Care Unit are springing up throughout the country. These differ considerably and, at the present time, no special guidelines can be laid down.

Until recently, most patients with AMI were discharged from the CCU to the general hospital, either to single, double, or quadruple semi-private rooms. No special attention was paid to the patients other than routine hospital care. All patients with myocardial infarction, either transmural or nontransmural in type, are now being discharged from the Coronary Care Unit to the Intermediate Coronary Care Unit. Patients who have been admitted to the hospital with suspected myocardial infarction, but who do not actually have such a disease, are discharged either to the general hospital or to home.

Description of ICCU

The Intermediate Coronary Care Unit consists of two rooms of four beds each for male patients and a two-bed room for female patients. All rooms are equipped with defibrillation apparatus, ECG machines, and resuscitation equipment. An ECG technician is assigned to take and mount rhythm strips every 4 hours. The strips, read immediately by a house officer, are kept as a permanent part of the chart. Remote telemetry is being installed in the ICCU to allow continuous display of ECG signals on the monitor bank of the main CCU. The Chief of Medicine or his representative is responsible for the movement of patients into and out of the unit. First priority is given to patients with transmural infarcts. Over 95 percent of coronary care patients are transferred to the ICCU on discharge from CCU. The essence of the ICCU, as with the CCU, is cardiac monitoring. The nurses here are also specially instructed in electrocardiography, cardiac arrhythmias, and cardiology.

Mortality Rate in ICCU

To date, 77 patients have been admitted to the ICCU, of whom 68 had a transmural infarction. The average duration in the CCU was 6 days. Based on the data in Fig. 2, Chapter 1, a further mortality of 10 deaths could be expected. Actually there were three deaths. Since the size of the series is small, no conclusion can be drawn from this experience. However, a favorable trend seems likely.

Complications
Developing in ICCU

Many complications developed in patients during their stay in the ICCU which were not present during the initial phase of their illness in the CCU. These are listed as follows:

Congestive heart failure	8
Arrhythmias	4
Extension of infarct	4
Psychosis	1
Pacemaker problems	1
Phlebitis	1

Congestive heart failure was controlled in all patients with digitalis and diuretic therapy. Of the four patients with arrhythmia, one was associated with an extension of infarction, one was controlled, and two patients expired. The arrhythmias encountered were transient atrial fibrillation, ventricular bigeminy, sinus bradycardia, conducted and non-conducted atrial premature beats, and complete and incomplete A-V dissociation. One episode of sinus bradycardia was associated with extension of an anterior infarct. The transient atrial fibrillation and the ventricular bigeminy, not associated with extension, were easily controlled by quinidine. Two deaths which were preceded by an arrhythmia are briefly reviewed:

CASE 1

A 56-year-old man was admitted 24 hours after the onset of chest pain, dizziness, syncope, and weakness. Serial electrocardiograms and serum enzymes were characteristic of an acute inferior wall myocardial infarction. Shortly after admission to the CCU, complete A-V dissociation appeared and a transvenous demand pacemaker was inserted. A Stokes-Adams attack due to ventricular fibrillation occurred on the 5th day. He was quickly defibrillated and recovered uneventfully. On the 11th day the pacemaker was removed, and he was transferred to the ICCU in regular sinus rhythm. The rhythm strip showed atrial premature beats, periods of isorhythmic dissociation, and junctional rhythm, all of which reverted spontaneously to sinus rhythm. On the 14th hospital day at 1 A.M., conducted and non-conducted atrial premature beats followed by long pauses were noted on the rhythm strip. The patient, examined almost immediately, was found to be pulseless, pale, and apneic. Resuscitation failed. Autopsy permission was refused.

CASE 2

A 56-year-old man with a long history of pulmonary tuberculosis was admitted with severe chest pain and diaphoresis of 24 hours duration. The presence of an acute anterior wall infarct was confirmed by ECG and serial enzymes. He developed a respiratory infection and congestive failure which responded to antibiotics, diuretics, and digitalis. On the 8th hospital day, much improved and still in sinus rhythm, he was transferred to the ICCU. The following night he was found pulseless and was immediately defibrillated with conversion to sinus rhythm. Multiple ventricular beats quickly appeared but were controlled with Lidocaine. Sinus rhythm then gave way to junctional rhythm which terminated in cardiac asystole. Intracardiac epinephrine produced ventricular fibrillation which could not be controlled and the patient expired. At autopsy there was a recent massive infarction of the left ventricular wall extending to the septum with early aneurysm and mural thrombus formation. A fresh embolus with infarction of the right lung was present along with old tuberculosis of both apices.

The third patient who died, expired at night suddenly and death was presumed to be due to an arrhythmia.

Methods of Cardiac Monitoring in ICCU

At the present time the role of the unit is far from settled. Two systems are being implemented: one in which the patient is continuously monitored by telemetry; and the other in which the patient has intermittent monitoring by the electrocardiograph machine, taking "rhythm strips" every 4 hours and having these mounted and read promptly. This latter practice is far short of ideal and represents an initial effort to detect arrhythmias as early as possible. When remote telemetry is operational, the patients in the ICCU, so far as arrhythmias are concerned, will be in the same protected environment as those in the CCU. Continuous observation will be possible, life-threatening arrhythmias will be anticipated or quickly recognized, and treatment will be prompt. The need for such a unit even with our presently limited facilities is apparent when we compare the three deaths that did occur with the 10 deaths expected from our previous experience on the general medical wards over the same period of time in acute transmural infarction.

References

Grace, W. J. and Yarvote, P. M. The intermediate coronary care unit —preliminary observations. Clin. Res., XVII, 4:579, 1969.

Most, A. S. and Peterson, D. R. Myocardial infarction surveillance. J.A.M.A., 208:2433, June 30, 1969.

Oliver, M. F., Julian, D. G., and Donald, K. W. Problems in evaluating coronary care units. Amer. J. Cardiol., 20:466, 1967.

Index